The Incidence and Economic Burden
of Injuries in the United States

The Incidence and Economic Burden of Injuries in the United States

Eric A. Finkelstein

Phaedra S. Corso

Ted R. Miller

and Associates

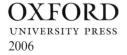
UNIVERSITY PRESS
2006

OXFORD
UNIVERSITY PRESS

Oxford University Press, Inc., publishes works that further
Oxford University's objective of excellence
in research, scholarship, and education.

Oxford New York
Auckland   Cape Town   Dar es Salaam   Hong Kong   Karachi
Kuala Lumpur   Madrid   Melbourne   Mexico City   Nairobi
New Delhi   Shanghai   Taipei   Toronto

With offices in
Argentina   Austria   Brazil   Chile   Czech Republic   France   Greece
Guatemala   Hungary   Italy   Japan   Poland   Portugal   Singapore
South Korea   Switzerland   Thailand   Turkey   Ukraine   Vietnam

Copyright © 2006 by Oxford University Press

Published by Oxford University Press, Inc.
198 Madison Avenue, New York, New York 10016

www.oup.com

Oxford is a registered trademark of Oxford University Press

Library of Congress Cataloging-in-Publication Data

Finkelstein, Eric
   The incidence and economic burden of injuries in the United States /
Eric A. Finkelstein, Phaedra S. Corso, Ted R. Miller, and Associates.
       p.   ; cm.
   Includes bibliographical references and index.
   ISBN-13 978-0-19-517948-4
   ISBN 0-19-517948-X
   1. Wounds and injuries—Economic aspects—United States. 2. Accidents—
Economic aspects—United States. 3. Wounds and injuries—United States—
Epidemiology. 4. Accidents—United States—Epidemiology.
   [DNLM: 1. Wounds and Injuries—economics—United States. 2. Accidents—
economics—United States. 3. Health Expenditures—United States.
4. Wounds and Injuries—epidemiology—United States. WO 700 F499i 2006]
I. Corso, Phaedra S.   II. Miller, Ted R.   III. Title.
   RD93.8.F56 2006
   614.30973—dc22   2005027736

9 8 7 6 5 4 3 2 1
Printed in the United States of America
on acid-free paper

Foreword

In looking forward to the 21st century, the Centers for Disease Control and Prevention identified both improved motor-vehicle safety and safer workplaces among the 10 greatest public health achievements of the last century. Indeed, death rates per million miles traveled have decreased an astonishing 90%, as have deaths per 100,000 workers. Despite these successes, injury remains the fourth leading cause of death over all ages and the leading cause of death and disability among our children and young adults. More young lives between the ages of 1 and 34 are lost to injury than to all other causes combined. And deaths due to injury only begin to tell the story. Injuries account for nearly 10% of all hospital discharges and more than one third of all emergency-department visits. Although many nonfatal injuries are minor in severity and result in only one or two days of restricted activity, a large proportion result in fractures, amputations, brain injuries, major burns, or other significant injuries that have far-reaching consequences for the individual, the family, the health care system, and society at large.

Now, for the first time in well over a decade, we have comprehensive estimates of the impact of these injuries in economic terms. The current volume builds significantly on work first published in 1989. Armed with more detailed and accurate data sources, together with improved coding and classification of injuries, the authors not only update previous figures but provide us with new estimates of cost by body region, and by nature and severity of injuries. Their work will become the new "must read" for anyone interested in reducing the burden of injury in our country.

These new estimates underscore the public health impact of injuries in terms of both health care costs and lost productivity. Injuries that occurred in 2000 will cost the U.S. health care system $80.2 billion in lifetime medical care costs. These high costs, however, are dwarfed by the costs associated with lost productivity resulting from premature death and disability. Injuries that occurred in 2000 will cost our society an estimated $326 billion in productivity losses: $142 billion for fatal injuries and $184 billion for nonfatal injuries.

While these figures are sobering, history has taught us that we can have an impact on their magnitude. But to do so we must continue to work together to further build the science of injury control and to make sure that the science is effectively translated into programs and policies that make a difference. Advances in primary and secondary prevention will be key to our overall success. But we must not lose sight of the difference effective treatment and rehabilitation can make in saving lives and promoting quality of life following the injuries we fail to prevent.

This incredibly rich compendium of data on the cost of injury will provide a much-needed resource to further this science by providing the tools to establish the value and return on investment of interventions that have been shown to be effective. For only by demonstrating the value of our interventions can we effectively advocate for their widespread implementation at the national, state, and local levels.

As we use these figures, however, we must remind ourselves that they describe the impact of injury in economic terms only. As such, they fail to communicate the often devastating consequences of injury on the personal lives of millions of people and their families. As we move forward in finding better ways of preventing injuries and ameliorating their consequences, we must not forget the personal stories behind them and what they can teach us.

Ellen J. MacKenzie, Ph.D.
Professor and Chair
Department of Health Policy & Management
Johns Hopkins Bloomberg School of Public Health

Preface

Injuries are one of the most serious public health problems facing the United States today. Through premature death, disability, medical costs and lost productivity, injuries significantly impact the health and welfare of Americans. Taken as a whole, injuries, both intentional and unintentional, are the leading cause of death among persons aged 1 to 44 years and the fourth leading cause of death among persons of all ages [Center for Disease Control and Prevention (CDC) Web-Based Injury Statistics Query and Reporting System (WISQARS) 2002]. Unlike other leading causes of death (e.g., tobacco use and poor diet/inactivity), however, deaths due to injuries affect the young and old alike. Because of this, the life-years lost due to injuries likely exceed those that result from other preventable causes.

Millions of Americans also suffer nonfatal injuries each year. Many of these injuries cause temporary discomfort but will not have lasting consequences. Other nonfatal injuries, however, will cause permanent losses in functional capacity. The health and economic burden of both temporary and permanent nonfatal injuries is substantial. All may entail significant medical treatment, reduced qualify of life, and lost productivity due to either temporary or permanent removal from the labor market.

Background

This book, *The Incidence and Economic Burden of Injuries in the United States,* provides a fresh look at the incidence and economic burden of injuries that occurred in 2000, including injury-attributable medical expenditures and the value of lost productivity resulting from these injuries. It updates the landmark study published by Dorothy Rice, Ellen MacKenzie, et al. in 1989. In their report to Congress, titled *Cost of Injury in the United States,* Rice and MacKenzie provided definitive lifetime cost estimates for injuries that occurred in 1985, stratified by age, sex, cause, and severity. The report became an instant "must read" for practitioners and researchers in injury prevention.

Rice and MacKenzie estimated that nearly one out of every four Americans was injured in 1985. These injuries resulted in 143,000 fatalities, 2.3 million hospitalizations, and 54 million nonhospitalized treatment episodes. The total economic costs of these injuries were estimated at $158 billion, or roughly $253 billion in 2000 dollars. Expenditures for medical care accounted for 29% of total costs, productivity losses accounted for 41% of total costs, and premature mortality accounted for 30% of total costs.

The 1989 report served as a methodological guide for a wide range of subsequent U.S.-based, injury-specific cost-of-illness analyses that uncovered costs such as the following: $5.8 billion for the costs of intimate partner violence in 1995 [CDC 2003]; $230.6 billion for the economic cost of motor vehicle crashes in 2000 [National Highway Traffic Safety Administration (NHTSA) 2002]; $81 billion for the economic cost of unintentional childhood injuries in 1996 [Miller et al. 2000]; and $40 billion for the economic cost of firearm injuries and $13 billion for the economic cost of cut/stab wounds in 1992 [Miller and Cohen 1997].

Since the 1989 report, however, no undertaking has addressed the incidence and economic burden of all injuries with more timely data, despite major changes in the field of prevention, reporting, and injury surveillance. For example, since 1985, new safety technologies (e.g., airbags in automobiles) have been developed to prevent injuries or to decrease the severity of injuries, and new policies and laws (e.g., state and local laws that require children to wear helmets when riding a bicycle) have been enacted to further promote injury prevention. Additionally, increases in mandatory reporting requirements (for suspected or confirmed child abuse cases, for example) exist in many jurisdictions, and new national surveys have been created that collect more complete surveillance information on injuries, costs, and productivity losses associated with injuries. These factors have the potential to influence either the prevalence and resulting cost of injuries since 1985, or our ability to accurately quantify these estimates.

The present book, funded under a contract from the National Center for Injury Prevention and Control (NCIPC) at the CDC, updates the 1989 report by using the best available data and methods. To accomplish this goal we convened a group of experts to discuss data sources and methodology for assessing incidence, and a second group to assess data sources and methodology for assessing costs. Participants included experts from academia, the federal government, and the private sector with considerable experience in injury control and prevention, epidemiology, national and state data sources, and economics. These experts provided input and feedback for every stage of study design and data analysis. A complete list of participants and other contributors to this book are included in the acknowledgments.

The estimates provided in this book describe the overall burden of injury in the United States. We define *burden* to include incidence, medical costs, productivity losses (i.e., wage and household work losses), and total costs (i.e., the sum of medical costs and the dollar value of productivity losses). *Incidence,* defined as the number of occurrences over a given time period, is often considered by the public health community when prioritizing burden. Burden, defined by medical expenditures to prevent illness and injury, is now also being considered, as health care costs continue to rise and increase the strain on public- and private-sector payers alike. Because, as noted above, the adverse effects of injuries are more likely to occur at younger ages relative to the adverse effects of smoking and other preventable diseases, productivity losses are likely to be the dominant cost associated with injuries. Inclusion of these losses is necessary for quantifying the true burden of injuries and for properly conducting cost-benefit analyses of injury-prevention activities.

As described in detail in the methods section of Chapter 1, the incidence of injuries, stratified across multiple dimensions (e.g., age, sex), is quantified using several data sources. Although many of these were not available in 1985, care was taken to apply a similar methodology to that used in the original study by Rice and MacKenzie. We applied the same definitions of injury and injury mechanisms, and stratified the estimates using identical age categories. Although undoubtedly some of the variation in incidence across the two studies will be due to methodological differences, these estimates provide the best source of information for comparing how the incidence of injuries has changed over the past 15 years, during which time many new technologies and initiatives aimed at reducing the overall burden of injuries were implemented.

To estimate the economic burden of injuries in this study, we conducted a cost-of-illness (COI) analysis [Rice 1966; Rice 1967; Hodgson and Meiners 1982; Rice et al. 1985]. A COI analysis, which can be either prevalence- or incidence-based, typically entails quantifying both the cost of medical treatment (direct) and the value of lost productivity (indirect). *Prevalence-based estimates* are cross-sectional estimates of costs that occur during a specified time period, typically a year, and are not dependent on when the illness first occurred [see Morbidity and Mortality Weekly Report (MMWR) 2004 for a prevalence-based annual estimate of the medical-care cost of injury]. In this book, as in the original study, we employ an incidence-based approach by quantifying the present value of lifetime costs that result from all injuries that occurred in the year 2000.

The COI estimates provided in this book can be used for several purposes. First, total cost estimates can be used to direct attention toward all injuries or a particular type of injury, serving to stimulate public policy debate concerning the appropriate funding level for injury prevention and research. Second, although some caveats apply, by comparing the 2000 cost estimates to those in the 1989 report, we can identify areas where injury-attributable costs have changed markedly over the past 15 years, perhaps due to changes in incidence, medical technology, or other causes. These trends, along with trends in incidence, may assist in determining both where prevention efforts have been successful and where additional prevention efforts are needed. Third, incidence-based estimates of injury-attributable costs can be used to establish the maximum amount of resources that could be saved through intervention efforts and are a necessary component of cost-effectiveness analyses (CEAs). Primers on how to use these methods for public health interventions have been described in detail elsewhere [Owens 2002; Haddix et al. 2003], some specifically detailing their application to injury and violence prevention [Miller and Levy 1997; Aos et al. 2001; Hornick et al. 2002]. Fourth, the scientific rigor employed in these analyses can serve as a methodological template for researchers interested in assessing COI estimates for other health outcomes of interest. All of these measures should prove invaluable to practitioners and researchers in injury prevention.

In summary, all four dimensions of burden (i.e., incidence, medical costs, productivity losses, and total costs) provide valuable information to practitioners, researchers, and policymakers. Depending on the issue being addressed, some or all of these dimensions of burden may be appropriate. A primary finding generated from this analysis is that the relative burden across injury mechanisms differs dramatically depending on which perspective is taken. For example, we show that motor vehicle accidents account for roughly 10% of the incidence of injuries but 22% of the total cost. Conversely, struck by/against injuries account for 22% of the incidence of injuries but only 12% of the total costs. These findings, along with other information on potential benefits of injury prevention activities, will assist policymakers in determining how best to allocate scarce research and prevention dollars.

Organization of the Book

This book contains five chapters on the incidence and economic burden of injuries. Chapter 1 provides estimates of the incidence of injuries in 2000 stratified by age, sex, mechanism, body region, nature of injury, and severity. Chapters 2 and 3 present lifetime medical costs and productivity losses, respectively, for these injuries using the same stratifications. Each of these chapters concludes with a section that describes the data and methods used in the analyses, and their limitations. Chapter 4 combines the medical and productivity losses to present the total lifetime costs of injuries in 2000 and presents a comparison of the relative burden of injuries across each of the dimensions presented in the previous chapters. Chapter 5 provides an overview of the results and discusses trends in incidence and costs by comparing our results to those reported in the 1989 report. It also includes a discussion of key limitations and areas for future injury research and prevention.

Acknowledgments

This report on the incidence and economic burden of injuries in the United States is the product of a 3-year research contract supported by the Centers for Disease Control and Prevention (CDC). It represents a collaborative effort between CDC, RTI International, and the Pacific Institute for Research and Evaluation (PIRE). The study involved a multitude of multidisciplinary experts, all of whom contributed greatly to the development of this report.

The authors gratefully acknowledge the participation of our expert panelists who provided invaluable contributions to the development of the overall study design and final peer review of results. Our sincere thanks to Ellen MacKenzie, Johns Hopkins; Lois Fingerhut, National Center for Health Statistics; Maria Segui-Gomez, University of Pamploma; Hank Weiss, University of Pittsburgh; Carol Runyan, University of North Carolina; Larry Blincoe, National Highway Traffic Safety Administration; Bill Zamula, Consumer Product Safety Commission; Steve Machlin, Agency for Healthcare Research and Quality; Wendy Max, University of California at San Francisco; and Scott Grosse, Renee Johnson, and Rick Waxweiler, CDC.

The principal investigators also acknowledge the professional expertise and assistance from several colleagues and support staff who had major responsibilities for the various components of the study. At RTI, Christian Gregory provided research assistance. At PIRE, Dexter Taylor conducted many of the analyses. At CDC, Lynda Doll and Ileana Arias provided technical expertise and policy guidance. Lee Annest, Linda Dahlberg, Jim Mercy, and David Sleet provided invaluable feedback on content and interpretation of results. And Bill Rhoads, Geetika Kalra, John Parmer, and Ram Shrestha did the editing.

We have enjoyed this collaborative effort both professionally and personally. Thank you for the opportunity.

Contents

The Incidence and Economic Burden of Injuries in the United States

Chapter 1

Incidence of Injuries in 2000

This chapter describes the number of injury episodes in 2000, how serious the injuries were, and the mechanism and nature of the injuries. Throughout, this chapter counts the number of injury episodes, meaning that if someone suffered multiple injuries (e.g., a leg fracture and an arm fracture) in one event (e.g., a fall), he or she would be counted only once; but if someone suffered the same two injuries in separate events on two different dates, he or she would be counted twice. For readability, this chapter often uses the terms *persons injured* or *number of injuries;* all the data presented, however, are on injury episodes.

As recommended by the International Collaborative Effort (ICE) on Injury Statistics and the State and Territorial Injury Prevention Director's Association (STIPDA), we considered the following International Classification of Diseases, 9th revision, Clinical Modification (ICD-9-CM) diagnoses as injuries: 800 through 909.2, 909.4, 909.9, 910 through 994.9, 995.5 through 995.59, and 995.80 through 995.85 (Injury Surveillance Workgroup, 2003). Diagnoses 905 through 909 (late effects of injury) and 958 (certain early complications of trauma) are excluded.

Estimated incidence counts and rates are presented for three mutually exclusive categories that reflect severity of injury: (1) injury resulting in death, including deaths occurring within and outside a health care setting; (2) injury resulting in hospitalization with survival to discharge; and (3) injuries that receive medical attention without hospitalization. The latter category includes injuries resulting in an emergency-department visit, an office-based visit, or a hospital outpatient visit. We sum "unduplicated" injuries across treatment settings to quantify total injuries. Injuries that are not medically attended are not included in this book.

For each injury category (i.e., fatal, hospitalized, nonhospitalized), incidence counts and rates were stratified by the following:

- Age and sex (for males and females in the following age categories: 0–4, 5–14, 15–24, 25–44, 45–64, 65–74, or 75 and older);
- Mechanism of injury (including motor vehicle/other road user, falls, struck by/ against, cut/pierce, fire/burn, poisoning, drowning/submersion, firearm/gunshot, or other);
- Body region (including traumatic brain injury, other head/neck, spinal cord injury, vertebral column injury, torso, upper extremity, lower extremity, other/unspecified, or system-wide based on the Barell Injury Diagnosis Matrix);
- Severity of injury (based on the Abbreviated Injury Score, [AIS]); and
- Nature of injury (including fracture, dislocation, sprain/strain, internal organ, open wound, amputation, blood vessel, superficial/contusion, crushing, burn, nerve, system-wide, or unspecified).

We do not stratify by race and ethnicity or place of injury because medical costs are not expected to vary along these dimensions. Although the data allow for a stratification by intent (e.g., unintentional, assault, self-inflicted, legal/military, undetermined), limitations in external cause coding (E codes) and reporting errors bias these estimates downward and so are not included in this book.

The estimates in this chapter were developed from multiple data sources, most with a base year of 2000; all results are therefore assumed to represent the incidence of injuries in 2000. Because of lack of availability, however, some data from 1999 and earlier were also used. Specifics regarding the methods and data used to develop these incidence estimates are detailed at the end of the chapter.

Total Injury Incidence

Table 1.1 displays incidence counts and rates for fatal, hospitalized, and nonhospitalized injuries by age and sex. In 2000, injuries in the United States resulted in approximately 149,000 fatalities, 1.9 million hospitalizations, and 48.1 million nonhospitalized treatment episodes. This sums to a total of 50.1 million injured persons, or 18 injured persons per every 100 U.S. civilian, noninstitutionalized residents.[1] In other words, almost one in five persons sustained an injury requiring medical attention (see the data and methods section at the end of this chapter for total population counts). As a fraction of all injuries, fatal injuries accounted for 0.3% of the total, hospitalized injuries accounted for 3.7%, and nonhospitalized injuries accounted for 95.9%.

The overall incidence of injuries among males (26.6 million) was only slightly higher than that among females (23.6 million). Taking into account population size, the overall rate of injuries for males was 20 per 100 persons and for females was

---

[1]For the denominator, we used the civilian, noninstitutionalized resident population provided in the 1999 Medical Expenditure Panel Survey (MEPS) to be consistent with our estimates of the incidence of nonfatal injuries derived from the same source. See the data and methods section at the end of this chapter.

Table 1.1 Incidence Counts and Rates (per 100,000) of Injuries by Age and Sex, 2000

Age Category and Sex	Fatal		Hospitalized		Nonhospitalized		Total	
	Incidence	Rate	Incidence	Rate	Incidence	Rate	Incidence	Rate
Total	*149,075*	*54*	*1,869,857*	*677*	*48,108,166*	*17,405*	*50,127,098*	*18,135*
0–4	3,532	18	47,203	240	3,375,836	17,145	3,426,571	17,403
5–14	3,741	9	88,432	214	7,853,619	19,025	7,945,792	19,249
15–24	23,698	63	218,437	585	8,576,279	22,956	8,818,414	23,604
25–44	48,487	59	434,710	526	15,069,810	18,233	15,553,007	18,818
45–64	31,935	53	337,373	565	8,445,245	14,132	8,814,553	14,750
65–74	10,595	60	189,079	1,072	2,179,600	12,356	2,379,274	13,488
75+	27,087	179	554,623	3,663	2,607,776	17,224	3,189,486	21,067
Male	*103,900*	*77*	*901,798*	*670*	*25,559,532*	*18,989*	*26,565,230*	*19,736*
0–4	2,059	20	27,283	266	2,049,692	19,958	2,079,034	20,244
5–14	2,397	11	56,590	270	4,482,442	21,406	4,541,429	21,688
15–24	18,609	98	141,990	748	4,968,976	26,180	5,129,575	27,026
25–44	37,126	92	272,739	676	8,243,991	20,446	8,553,856	21,215
45–64	23,313	81	183,324	634	4,002,098	13,843	4,208,735	14,558
65–74	6,916	87	73,816	924	974,981	12,204	1,055,713	13,215
75+	13,480	228	146,057	2,465	837,352	14,134	996,889	16,827
Female	*45,175*	*32*	*968,059*	*683*	*22,548,634*	*15,902*	*23,561,868*	*16,616*
0–4	1,473	16	19,921	212	1,326,144	14,083	1,347,538	14,311
5–14	1,344	7	31,842	157	3,371,177	16,574	3,404,363	16,737
15–24	5,089	28	76,447	416	3,607,303	19,616	3,688,839	20,059
25–44	11,361	27	161,971	383	6,825,819	16,125	6,999,151	16,535
45–64	8,622	28	154,049	499	4,443,147	14,402	4,605,818	14,930
65–74	3,679	38	115,263	1,194	1,204,619	12,479	1,323,561	13,711
75+	13,607	148	408,566	4,432	1,770,424	19,204	2,192,597	23,783

17 per 100 persons. Of the total injuries in 2000, almost one third (15.6 million) occurred among 25- to 44-years-old. This is not surprising, however, given that this age group also represents approximately one third of the U.S. population. In comparison, 15- to 24-year-olds represent only 14% of the U.S. population but accounted for 18% of injuries. Because of this, 15- to 24-year-olds, with 8.8 million injuries, had the highest *rate* of injuries, 24 per 100 persons; the second-highest rate, 21 per 100 persons, occurred among those aged 75 years and older; and the third-highest rate, 19 per 100 persons, occurred among those aged 5 to 14 years. These high injury rates across different age groups reveal that, unlike chronic conditions (e.g., heart disease, diabetes, osteoarthritis), which disproportionately affect the elderly, injuries affect both the young and old alike. It follows, as we show in chapters 2 and 3, that the economic burden of injuries is much larger than that for many chronic conditions because injuries are more likely to impact people during their peak earning years.

Figure 1.1 illustrates the rate of injury episodes per 100,000 persons by age and sex. The relatively balanced distribution across these diverse populations reflects the wide-ranging impact of injuries on public health. For those age groups with persons

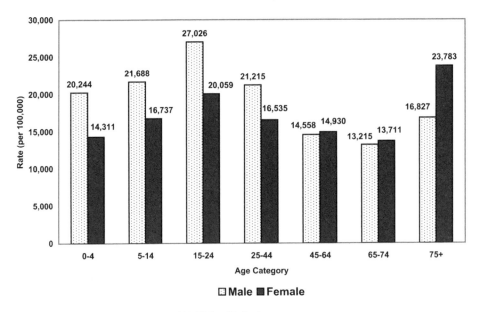

Figure 1.1 Incidence Rates (per 100,000) of Injuries

younger than 44 years, males had a higher rate of injuries than females; however, for those age groups with persons older than 45 years, females had a higher rate of injuries. The highest rate of injuries for males, 27 per 100 persons, occurred among those aged 15 to 24 years. The highest rate of injuries for females, 24 per 100 persons, occurred among females aged 75 years and older. The following section further examines injuries by age and sex patterns, taking into account severity (i.e., fatal, hospitalized, nonhospitalized injuries).

Age and Sex Patterns

For fatal injuries, the highest incidence (48,000, or 32%) occurred among those persons aged 25 to 44 years old (Table 1.1). This was true for both males (37,000, or 36%) and females (11,000, or 25%). An examination of the incidence of fatal injuries by age and sex reveals that males had a higher incidence of fatal injuries than females for all age groups with the exception of those aged 75 years and older.

The highest rate of injury fatalities, 179 per 100,000, occurred among persons aged 75 years and older (Table 1.1), and was nearly 3 times greater than the next highest rate, 63 per 100,000, which occurred among persons 15 to 24 years old. Further stratifying the rate of fatal injuries by sex indicates that males in every age group were more likely to suffer a fatal injury than their female counterparts (Figure 1.2). In fact, the overall rate of injury fatalities among males (77 per 100,000 persons) was more than double that among females (32 per 100,000 persons).

Not only did persons 75 years and older have the highest rate of fatal injuries, they also had the highest rate of hospitalized injuries (Figure 1.3). Persons aged 75 years

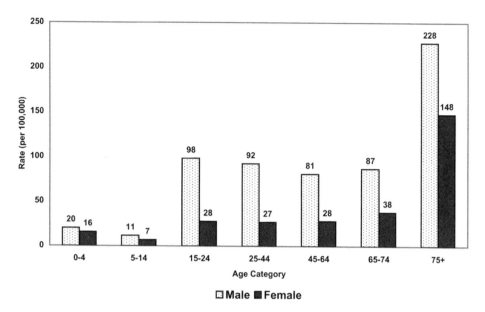

Figure 1.2 Incidence Rates (per 100,000) of Fatal Injuries

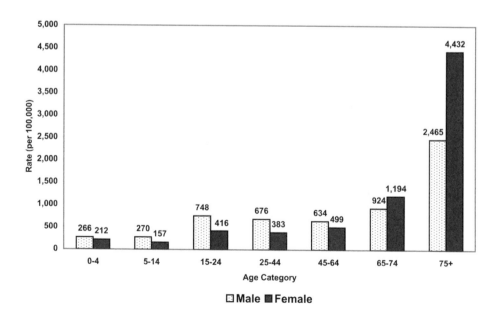

Figure 1.3 Incidence Rates (per 100,000) of Hospitalized Injuries

and older accounted for nearly 555,000 injury hospitalizations, or 30% of the total (Table 1.1). Because this age group makes up such a small fraction of the U.S. population (3%), its rate of injury hospitalizations, 3.7 per 100 persons, is more than 3 times that of any other age group. For males, although the highest number of injury hospitalizations (273,000, or 30%) occurred among those 25 to 44 years old, the highest *rate* of injury hospitalizations (2.5 per 100 persons) occurred among those aged 75 years and older (Figure 1.3). For females, both the highest number (409,000, or 42%) and the highest rate of injury hospitalizations occurred among those aged 75 years and older. In fact, the rate of injury hospitalizations (4.4 per 100 persons) among elderly females was nearly 4 times greater than that among any other female age group.

Patterns of injury by age and sex are considerably different for less severe injuries (i.e., injuries not resulting in death or hospitalization). Unlike fatal and hospitalized injuries, nonhospitalized injuries are more likely to occur among the younger populations. Males and females 25 to 44 years old, who represent 30% of the total population, had the highest incidence of nonhospitalized injuries (Table 1.1). The highest *rate* of nonhospitalized injuries, however, occurred among persons 15 to 24 years old (Figure 1.4). Among this group, nonhospitalized injury rates were 26.2 injuries per 100 males and 19.6 injuries per 100 females.

Mechanism of Injuries

A critical step in injury prevention is to understand the mechanisms or sources of injuries. As shown in Table 1.2, the distribution of injuries by mechanism categories varies considerably for fatal, hospitalized, and nonhospitalized injuries. The two

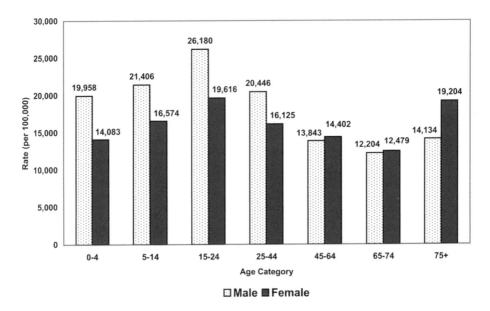

Figure 1.4 Incidence Rates (per 100,000) of Nonhospitalized Injuries

Table 1.2 Incidence Counts and Rates (per 100,000) of Injuries by Mechanism and Sex, 2000

Mechanism and Sex	Fatal		Hospitalized		Nonhospitalized		Total	
	Incidence	Rate	Incidence	Rate	Incidence	Rate	Incidence	Rate
Total	*149,075*	*54*	*1,869,857*	*676*	*48,108,166*	*17,405*	*50,127,098*	*18,135*
MV/other road user	43,802	16	276,183	100	4,690,454	1,697	5,010,439	1,813
Falls	14,052	5	854,589	309	10,698,101	3,870	11,566,742	4,185
Struck by/against	1,301	0	85,687	31	10,587,192	3,830	10,674,180	3,862
Cut/pierce	2,293	1	71,129	26	4,050,663	1,465	4,124,085	1,492
Fire/burn	3,922	1	24,519	9	745,935	270	774,376	280
Poisoning	20,261	7	219,056	79	1,028,148	372	1,267,465	459
Drowning/submersion	4,168	2	3,289	1	2,626	1	10,083	4
Firearm/gunshot	28,722	10	29,609	11	72,682	26	131,013	47
Other	30,554	11	305,796	111	16,232,366	5,873	16,568,716	5,994
Male	*103,900*	*77*	*901,798*	*670*	*25,559,533*	*18,989*	*26,565,232*	*19,736*
MV/other road user	29,686	22	167,893	125	2,353,751	1,749	2,551,330	1,895
Falls	7,647	6	306,583	228	4,887,446	3,631	5,201,676	3,865
Struck by/ against	1,109	1	66,833	50	6,592,359	4,898	6,660,301	4,948
Cut/Pierce	1,678	1	50,354	37	2,550,052	1,895	2,602,084	1,933
Fire/Burn	2,333	2	15,069	11	354,586	263	371,988	276
Poisoning	13,721	10	90,090	67	485,089	360	588,900	438
Drowning/submersion	3,198	2	2,166	2	1,652	1	7,016	5
Firearm/gunshot	24,638	18	26,278	20	66,113	49	117,029	87
Other	19,890	15	176,532	131	8,268,486	6,143	8,464,908	6,289
Female	*45,175*	*32*	*968,059*	*683*	*22,548,634*	*15,902*	*23,561,868*	*16,616*
MV/other road user	14,116	10	108,289	76	2,336,703	1,648	2,459,108	1,734
Falls	6,405	5	548,006	386	5,810,655	4,098	6,365,066	4,489
Struck by/against	192	0	18,855	13	3,994,833	2,817	4,013,880	2,831
Cut/Pierce	615	0	20,775	15	1,500,611	1,058	1,522,001	1,073
Fire/Burn	1,589	1	9,450	7	391,349	276	402,389	284
Poison	6,540	5	128,966	91	543,059	383	678,565	479
Drowning/submersion	970	1	1,123	1	974	1	3,067	2
Firearm/gunshot	4,084	3	3,331	2	6,569	5	13,984	10
Other	10,664	8	129,263	91	7,963,880	5,616	8,103,807	5,715

leading mechanisms of fatal injuries were motor vehicles and firearms, accounting for 43,802 and 28,722 deaths, respectively (or 16 and 10 per 100,000 persons, respectively). These two mechanisms were responsible for nearly half (49%) of all injury fatalities. In contrast, falls caused both the highest number (854,600, or 46%) and rate of hospitalized injuries (309 per 100,000 persons). In fact, the rate of fall-related hospitalized injuries was more than 3 times greater than any other specified mechanism category. Motor vehicles (276,200, or 15%) and poisonings (219,000, or 12%) represented the second and third leading mechanisms of hospitalized injuries, respectively. For nonhospitalized injuries, falls (10.7 million) and being struck by or against an object (10.6 million) were the most likely injury mechanisms, at a comparable rate of 3.8 per 100 persons.

Injuries categorized as "other" resulted from varied mechanisms. For fatal injuries, these other mechanisms, representing 20% of the total, included inhalation/suffocation (8% of all deaths) and unspecified (8%). Hospitalized injuries resulting from other mechanisms were largely related to unspecified mechanisms (5%), other transport (2%), and overexertion (2%); they represented 16% of all hospitalized injuries. For less severe nonhospitalized injuries, other mechanisms represented 34% of the total, with the largest contributors being overexertion (11%), bite/sting (7%), and other transport (2%).

Examining mechanism by sex, males had a higher incidence of injuries for all categories except falls, fire/burns, and poisoning. Of all fall-related injuries, 55% occurred among females, a rate of 4.5 per 100 females. This rate is 15% higher than the rate of fall injuries among males (3.9 per 100 persons). However, the most substantial difference between males and females occurred for firearm/gunshot-related injuries, with males suffering 89% of these injuries. The rate of firearm injuries among males, 87 per 100,000 persons, was almost 9 times that among females, 10 per 100,000 persons.

Largely because of firearm-/gunshot-related injuries, which tend to be more severe, males accounted for the majority of injury fatalities, nearly 70%, despite the fact that they represent only 49% of the total population (see the data and methods section at the end of this chapter for total population counts). As shown in Table 1.2, males had a higher incidence of fatal injuries, regardless of mechanism category. Similarly, the rates of fatal injuries by mechanism were all higher for males than for females. This difference was particularly pronounced for motor-vehicle-related and firearm-related fatal injuries. The rate of fatal motor-vehicle-related injuries among males (22 per 100,000 persons) was more than double that among females (10 per 100,000 persons); the rate of fatal firearm injuries among males (18 per 100,000 persons) was 6 times that among females (3 per 100,000 persons).

Although females accounted for 52% of all hospitalized injuries, males had higher incidence counts and rates for all mechanisms other than falls and poisonings (Table 1.2). Females accounted for 548,000 (64%) and 129,000 (58%) of fall- and poisoning-related hospitalized injuries, respectively. The rate of fall-related hospitalized injuries among females (386 per 100,000 persons) was 69% higher than that among males (228 per 100,000). Males, on the other hand, accounted for more than 70% of struck by-/against- (78%), cut-/pierce- (71%), and firearm-/gunshot-related (89%) hospitalized injuries. The rate of firearm-/gunshot-related hospitalized injuries among males (20 per 100,000 persons) was 10 times higher than that among females (2 per 100,000 persons).

The distribution of nonhospitalized injuries by mechanism resembles the distribution of fatal and hospitalized injuries by mechanism. Males accounted for the overwhelming majority of nonhospitalized firearm/gunshot injuries (66,000, or 90%), while females accounted for more than 54% of fall-related nonhospitalized injuries. The rate of nonhospitalized firearm-/gunshot-related injuries among males, 49 per 100,000 persons, was almost 10 times that among females, 5 per 100,000 persons. The rate of nonhospitalized fall injuries among females, 4 per 100 persons, was 10% greater than the rate among males, 3.6 per 100 persons.

Injuries by Body Region, Severity, and Nature of Injury

Information about the medical nature of injuries and the severity, or threat to life, they pose primarily serves people interested in treatment planning and recovery prospects. Figure 1.5 shows the breakdown of injuries by severity. Severity is measured by AIS score, a scale that bases its threat-to-life estimates primarily on the nature and degree of damage to different body regions. It ranges from 1, a minor injury with a high likelihood of survival, to 6, an injury that is virtually unsurvivable. We computed the AIS scores shown. In cases where individuals experience multiple injuries (which is common in motor vehicle crashes, for example), we categorize the injury based on the highest AIS severity level among all individual injuries (see the data and methods section at the end of this chapter for more information). As illustrated in Figure 1.5, nearly 85% of injuries were minor or moderate (AIS 1 or 2), and the majority of the remaining injuries (13.9%) were of unknown severity because it could not be coded from diagnoses alone without, for example, information on Glascow Coma Scale scores or on blood volume lost that does not appear in discharge records. Only 1.6% of injuries were coded as serious (AIS 3), 0.3% were severe (AIS 4), and 0.1% were critical (AIS 5).

Table 1.3 shows the distribution of total injuries by body region. Injuries to upper and lower extremities were by far the most frequent, comprising 27% and 22% of all injuries, respectively. Injuries to the head and neck (other than traumatic brain injury) occurred in 13% of injuries. For fatal injuries, traumatic brain injuries accounted for 27%, system-wide injuries for 26%, and injuries to the torso for 15%. For hospitalized injuries, 35% were to the lower extremities, 15% were system-wide, and 15% were to upper extremities. For nonhospitalized injuries, upper and lower extremities comprised 27% and 22% of the total, respectively, while nontraumatic head injury comprised 13% of nonhospitalized injuries.

The distribution of nonfatal injury incidence by severity (represented by AIS score) and body region is displayed in Table 1.4. For minor and moderate injuries

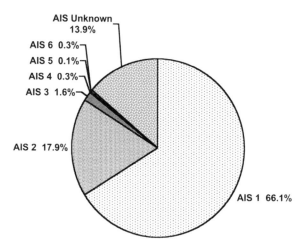

Figure 1.5 Injuries by Severity

Table 1.3 Incidence Counts and Rates (per 100,000) of Injuries by Body Region, 2000

Body Region	Fatal		Hospitalized		Nonhospitalized		Total	
	Incidence	Rate	Incidence	Rate	Incidence	Rate	Incidence	Rate
Total	*149,075*	*54*	*1,869,857*	*676*	*48,108,166*	*17,405*	*50,127,098*	*18,135*
Traumatic Brain Injury	40,148	15	155,587	56	1,147,485	415	1,343,220	486
Other Head/Neck	4,602	2	144,085	52	6,391,816	2,312	6,540,502	2,366
Spinal Cord Injury	759	0	10,316	4	15,987	6	27,062	10
Vertebral Column Injury	767	0	86,218	31	4,618,826	1,671	4,705,811	1,702
Torso	23,124	8	244,651	89	3,887,527	1,406	4,155,302	1,503
Upper Extremity	885	0	275,304	100	13,047,368	4,720	13,323,556	4,820
Lower Extremity	7,340	3	656,201	237	10,583,952	3,829	11,247,492	4,069
Other/Unspecified	32,365	12	18,365	7	5,788,736	2,094	5,839,466	2,113
System-wide	39,085	14	279,131	101	2,626,469	950	2,944,686	1,065

(AIS 1 and 2), upper and lower extremities accounted for 30% and 25%, respectively. For serious injuries (AIS 3), lower extremities accounted for 57%, injuries to the torso accounted for 22%, and injuries to the upper extremities accounted for 6%. For severe injuries (AIS 4), 75% were traumatic brain injuries, 18% were torso injuries, and 2% were spinal cord injuries. Critical injuries (AIS 5) most frequently occurred to the torso (31%), the brain (28%), and the upper extremities (24%).

Fifty-three percent of all hospitalizations were for minor or moderate injuries (AIS 1 and 2), with 32% involving the lower extremities, 25% involving the upper extremities, and 13% involving the torso. Nearly 67% of all serious (AIS 3) hospitalized injuries involved the lower extremities, with the torso and upper extremities involved in an additional 18% and 5% of serious hospitalized injuries, respectively. Of the 78,000 hospitalized injuries that were severe (AIS 4), traumatic brain injuries made up 75%. Of the 14,000 critical (AIS 5) injury hospitalizations, the highest incidence counts were for traumatic brain injury (52%), injuries to the torso (35%), and spinal cord injuries (9%).

The most common injuries by nature, as shown in Figure 1.6, were sprains and strains, which accounted for 30% of all injuries, or approximately 15 million injury episodes (incidence counts are represented in Appendix Table 1.1). Superficial injuries/contusions accounted for 21% (or 10.5 million) and open wounds for 18% (or 8.9 million). Fractures accounted for another 14% (or 7 million).

As Appendix Table 1.2 shows, of injuries with specified nature, system-wide injuries accounted for 26% of all fatal injuries. Fractures were the most frequent hospitalized injury, comprising 49% of the total. Sprains and strains made up the greatest fraction of nonhospitalized injury, accounting for 31% of the total.

Patterns of Injuries by Mechanism

The following section details incidence counts and rates of injury by mechanism, with stratifications by age and gender. Incidence counts and rates referred to below are detailed in Appendix Tables 1.3 through 1.11.

Table 1.4 Incidence Counts and Rates (per 100,000) of Nonfatal Injuries by Body Region and Severity, 2000

Body Region	AIS*	Hospitalized		Nonhospitalized		Total	
		Incidence	Rate	Incidence	Rate	Incidence	Rate
Total		*1,869,857*	*676*	*48,108,166*	*17,405*	*49,978,023*	*18,081*
Traumatic brain	1	10,114	4	33,072	12	43,186	16
injury	2	44,634	16	267,942	97	312,576	113
	3	21,975	8	20,095	7	42,070	15
	4	59,155	21	39,611	14	98,766	36
	5	7,326	3	0	0	7,326	3
	Unknown	12,588	5	147,012	53	159,600	58
Other head/neck	1	110,075	40	6,251,319	2,262	6,361,394	2,301
	2	25,079	9	201,552	73	226,631	82
	3	5,355	2	10,080	4	15,436	6
	4	1,557	1	0	0	1,557	1
	5	141	0	0	0	141	0
	Unknown	2,040	1	569,574	206	571,614	207
Spinal cord injury	1	93	0	0	0	93	0
	2	93	0	0	0	93	0
	3	5,239	2	10,745	4	15,984	6
	4	3,066	1	0	0	3,066	1
	5	1,337	0	0	0	1,337	0
	Unknown	528	0	5,242	2	5,770	2
Vertebral column	1	14,963	5	4,403,136	1,593	4,418,098	1,598
injury	2	65,751	24	188,610	68	254,362	92
	3	3,267	1	0	0	3,267	1
	4	617	0	1,872	1	2,489	1
	5	103	0	2,683	1	2,785	1
	Unknown	1,363	0	23,112	8	24,475	9
Torso	1	58,610	21	3,127,845	1,132	3,186,454	1,153
	2	68,213	25	160,827	58	229,040	83
	3	88,085	32	80,921	29	169,005	61
	4	11,664	4	12,081	4	23,745	9
	5	4,894	2	3,103	1	7,996	3
	Unknown	12,783	5	502,294	182	515,077	186
Upper extremity	1	98,322	36	9,144,995	3,308	9,243,317	3,344
	2	148,075	54	3,382,272	1,224	3,530,347	1,277
	3	24,213	9	26,024	9	50,237	18
	4	814	0	0	0	814	0
	5	101	0	6,143	2	6,244	2
	Unknown	3,089	1	489,423	177	492,512	178
Lower extremity	1	80,764	29	5,924,257	2,143	6,005,021	2,173
	2	237,872	86	4,094,520	1,481	4,332,392	1,567
	3	329,693	119	115,940	42	445,633	161
	4	1,898	1	0	0	1,898	1
	5	240	0	0	0	240	0
	Unknown	5,834	2	450,323	163	456,156	165
Other/unspecified	1	12,072	4	3,702,630	1,340	3,714,702	1,344
	2	1,347	0	62,379	23	63,727	23
	3	436	0	34,823	13	35,260	13
	4	24	0	0	0	24	0

continued

Table 1.4 *Continued*

Body Region	AIS*	Hospitalized		Nonhospitalized		Total	
		Incidence	Rate	Incidence	Rate	Incidence	Rate
	5	21	0	0	0	21	0
	Unknown	5,205	2	1,985,244	718	1,990,449	720
System-wide	1	6,003	2	157,131	57	163,135	59
	2	3,052	1	0	0	3,052	1
	3	439	0	0	0	439	0
	4	65	0	0	0	65	0
	5	4	0	0	0	4	0
	Unknown	269,569	98	2,469,338	893	2,738,907	991

*AIS Score for fatal injuries not available.

Motor-Vehicle/Other Road-User Injuries

Motor vehicle and other road users (which includes motor-vehicle occupants, motorcyclists, pedalcyclists, pedestrians, and motor-vehicle transport unspecified) were the leading mechanism of injury death, resulting in 43,802 deaths in 2000 (see Table 1.2). They also comprise the second leading mechanism of injury hospitalizations (276,183) and the third leading mechanism of less severe, nonhospitalized injuries (4.7 million). Of the 5 million motor-vehicle and other road-user injured victims in 2000, 68% were suffered by motor-vehicle occupants, 13% by pedalcyclists, 5% by those on motorcycles, and 4% by pedestrians (Appendix Table 1.3).

Adolescents and young adults aged 15 to 24 were at the highest risk of both fatal and nonfatal injuries related to motor-vehicles and other road-user injuries (Figure

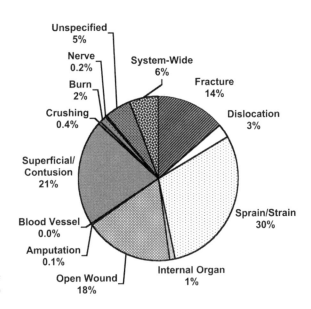

Figure 1.6 Injuries by Nature of Injury, 2000

1.7). Figure 1.8 shows the rates of fatal motor-vehicle injury by age group and gender. For both males and females, those older than 75 years had the highest rate of motor-vehicle fatalities (43 per 100,000 for men and 23 per 100,000 for women), followed by those aged 15 to 24 years (41 per 100,000 for men and 17 per 100,000 for women). Over age 15, males were almost twice as likely as females to die from a motor-vehicle crash, with the largest male to female ratio (3-fold) observed in the 25 to 44 age group.

Males are also more likely to be hospitalized as a result of a motor-vehicle injury, although the sex differential is not as great as for fatalities (Figure 1.9). For those aged 15 to 24 years, the rate of hospitalized motor-vehicle-related injuries among males, 216 per 100,000, was 80% higher than the rate among females of this same age, at 120 per 100,000. For those aged 25 to 44 years, the rate of hospitalized motor-vehicle-related injury for males, 147 per 100,000, was 93% greater than the rate for females, at 76 per 100,000.

A somewhat different pattern is observed for minor, nonhospitalized injuries. As shown in Figure 1.10, the rate of treatment for nonhospitalized motor-vehicle-related injury for males was higher than the rate for females for those aged 0 to 14, 25 to 44, and 75 years old and older. In contrast, females 15 to 24 and 45 to 74 had slightly higher rates than same-aged males.

Fortunately, motor-vehicle injuries are largely preventable. Since 1966, the United States has witnessed a 73% reduction in motor-vehicle death rates (per 100,000,000 vehicle miles) under the leadership of the Department of Transportation and De-

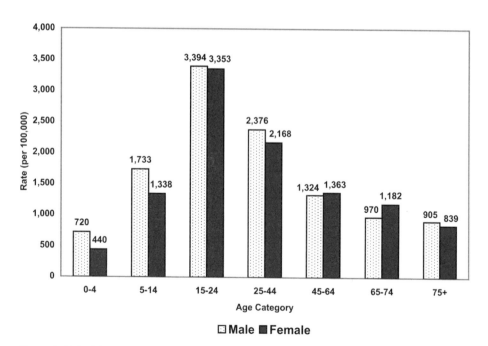

Figure 1.7 Incidence Rate (per 100,000) of Motor-Vehicle/Other Road-User Injuries

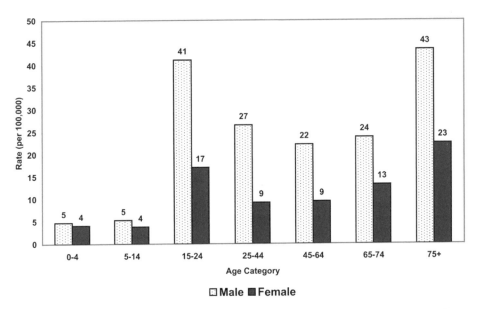

Figure 1.8 Incidence Rate (per 100,000) of Fatal Motor-Vehicle/Other Road-User Injuries

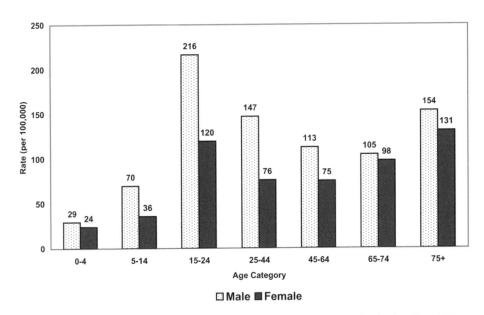

Figure 1.9 Incidence Rate (per 100,000) of Hospitalized Motor-Vehicle/Other Road-User Injuries

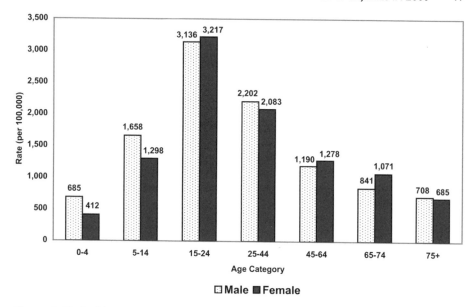

Figure 1.10 Incidence Rate (per 100,000) of Nonhospitalized Motor-Vehicle/Other Road-User Injuries

partment of Health and Human Services, and guidelines set forth in the Federal Motor Vehicle Safety Standards [National Safety Council 2003; CDC 1999]. These reductions were the result of research and program activities combined with enactment and enforcement of traffic safety laws, changes in vehicle and highway design, public education, and changes in driver and passenger behavior. Addressing issues such as speeding, impaired driving, helmet use, seat belts and child passenger restraints, visibility of cyclists and pedestrians, road design, enforcement of road safety regulations, reductions in traffic exposure, and improved emergency response can all work to further reduce deaths and injuries from motor-vehicle injuries in the United States and throughout the world [CDC 1999; Peden et al. 2004; Dellinger et al. 2005].

Falls

Falls, which are mostly unintentional, were the leading mechanism of hospitalized injuries in the United States in 2000, accounting for 854,589 hospitalizations (see Table 1.2). They also comprised the leading mechanism of less severe nonhospitalizations (10.7 million) and caused 14,052 deaths.

The overall distribution of rates of fall injuries by age and gender suggests that fall injuries had a substantial effect on all age groups, but the young and old in particular. The distribution follows a u-shaped pattern, with the lowest rates among males 45 to 64 years old and among females 15 to 24 years old, and the highest rates on the lower and upper ends of the age distribution for each gender, respectively (Figure 1.11).

Fatal fall rates are higher among males than females. The underlying causes for this gender difference are unclear. Males may sustain more severe injuries than

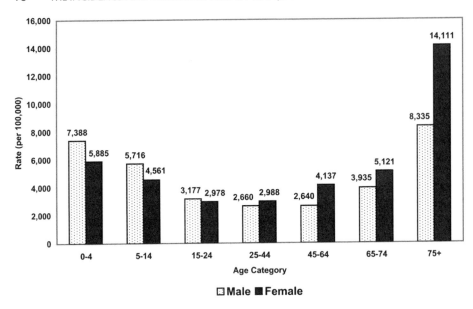

Figure 1.11 Incidence Rate (per 100,000) of Fall Injuries

females because they fall from greater heights, such as from ladders. Or, males may have more underlying chronic conditions than females of comparable age, be in poorer health, and be less able to survive a fall-related injury.

Unlike fatal fall rates, hospitalized and nonhospitalized fall injury rates are higher among older females (Figure 1.12 and Figure 1.13). To some extent, this may reflect gender differences in levels of physical activity [Davis 1994]. Muscle weakness and loss of lower-body strength, often caused by inactivity, are well-known risk factors for falling [American Geriatrics Society 2001]. Differences in physical activity levels also may influence the circumstances or events contributing to females' higher injury rate, as well as help explain their lower mortality.

The elderly are at the highest risk of dying and/or being hospitalized as the result of a fall. The rate of falls resulting in death among the elderly was more than 5 times greater than for any other age group among both males and females, and the risk of hospitalization was more than 3 times as great. Falls among older adults are a major health problem. More than a third of older adults fall each year [Hornbrook 1994; Hausdorff 2001] and fall-related injuries cause significant mortality, disability, and loss of independence [Sterling 2001]. Falls are the leading cause of unintentional injury death among older adults. Osteoporosis, which is a widespread disease among older women and which increases in prevalence as a person ages, greatly increases the chance a person who falls will suffer a hip fracture [Melton 1992; Greenspan 1994].

A slightly different pattern is observed for falls resulting in less severe, nonhospitalized injuries (Figure 1.14). Females aged 75 years and older remained the highest risk; they accounted for 10,285 injuries per 100,000 persons. However, children less than 15 years of age were also at high risk; they comprised the next highest age group at risk for minor injury due to falls.

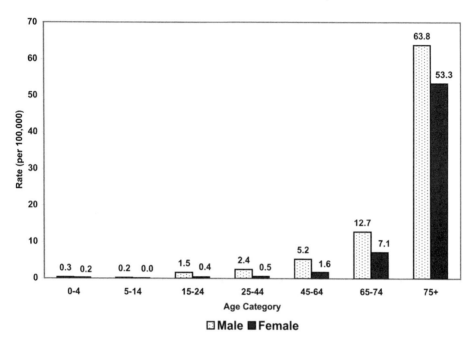

Figure 1.12 Incidence Rate (per 100,000) of Fatal Fall Injuries

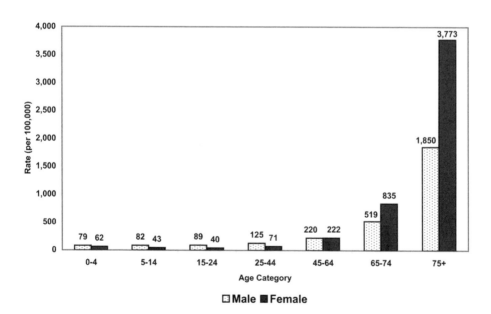

Figure 1.13 Incidence Rate (per 100,000) of Hospitalized Fall Injuries

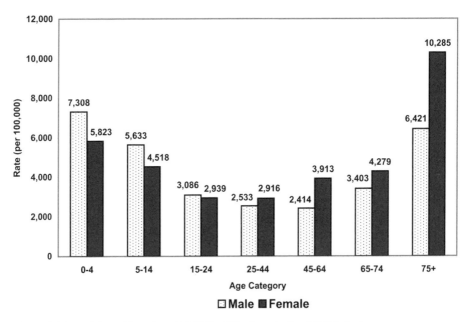

Figure 1.14 Incidence Rate (per 100,000) of Nonhospitalized Fall Injuries

In recent years, a number of systematic reviews have evaluated intervention strategies to determine what works [Scott 2001; Gillespie 2002; RAND 2003; Gillespie 2004; Hill 2004]. The Rand Report [RAND 2003] concluded that fall prevention programs as a group effectively reduced the risk of falling by 11%. Effective prevention strategies included clinical assessment combined with individualized fall risk reduction and patient follow-up; exercise to improve balance and strength; and reducing the number and types of medications used if possible, particularly tranquilizers, sleeping pills, and anti-anxiety drugs. Multi-component interventions use a combination of strategies to reduce fall risk factors. These included risk-factor screening; tailored exercise or physical therapy to improve gait, balance, and strength; medication management; and other elements such as education about fall risk factors, referrals to health care providers for treatment of chronic conditions that may contribute to fall risk, and having vision assessed and corrected [Close 1999; McMurdo 2000; Day 2002; Nikolaus 2003; Clemson 2004]. Home assessment and modification was most useful when it was combined with other strategies.

Struck by/against

Injuries classified as struck by/against include those resulting from being struck by (hit) or crushed by a human, animal, or inanimate object or force other than a vehicle or machinery, and those caused by striking (hitting) against a human, animal, or inanimate object or force other than a vehicle or machinery. While struck by/against injuries were the second leading mechanism of nonhospitalized injuries (10.6 million), they accounted for the lowest incidence of injury deaths (1,301) (see Table 1.2).

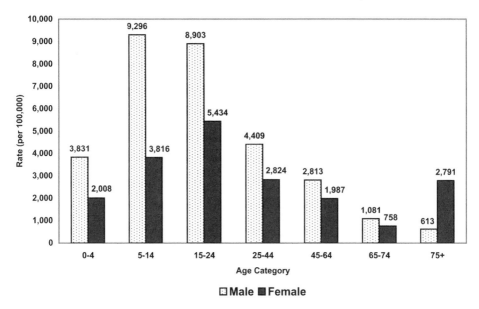

Figure 1.15 Incidence Rate (per 100,000) of Struck by/against Injuries

Figure 1.15 shows the incidence rates of struck by/against injury by age and gender. It shows that males 5 to 14 years old had the highest rate of struck by/against injury, nearly 2 times greater than the rate for any other female age category. Overall, males had higher rates of injury in all age groups except for persons aged 75 years and older, where the rate for females was more than 4 times the rate for males.

The incidence rates of hospitalized struck by/against injuries were much higher for males than for females, with the exception of the elderly (Figure 1.16). At 15 to 24 years of age, when the rate of hospitalized struck-by/against injury peaks for males, their rate (87 per 100,000 males) was nearly 6 times greater than the rate for females (15 per 100,000 females). Incidence for females peaked among those 75 years and older, yet the rate was comparable to the rate among same-aged males.

The rates for nonhospitalized injuries, which accounted for 99% of the incidence of struck by/against injuries, followed a similar pattern (Figure 1.17). The rates were higher for males than females for all age groups except the elderly. At 5 to 14 years of age, when the rate of nonhospitalized struck by/against injury peaked for males, their rate was more than 2 times greater than the rate for females. Incidence for females peaked among those 75 years and over at nearly 5 times greater than the rate for same-aged males.

Cut/Pierce

Injuries due to cutting or piercing instruments or objects (e.g., lawnmowers, knives, stiff paper, rocks) accounted for 4.1 million injuries; the vast majority of these (98%) did not result in a fatality or hospital admission.

Figure 1.18 shows the rate of cut/pierce injury by age and gender. Males less than 45 years of age had a higher incidence of cut/pierce injury than females, with the

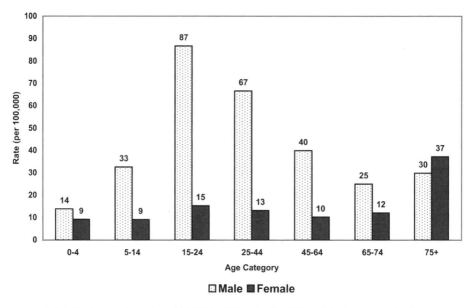

Figure 1.16 Incidence Rate (per 100,000) of Hospitalized Struck by/against Injuries

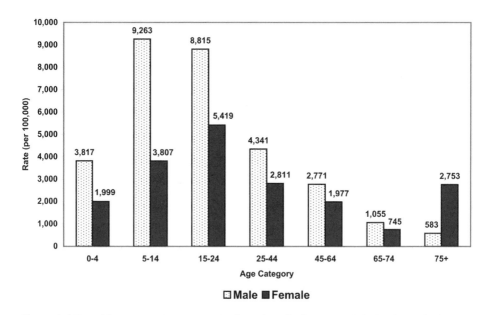

Figure 1.17 Incidence Rate (per 100,000) of Nonhospitalized Struck by/against Injuries

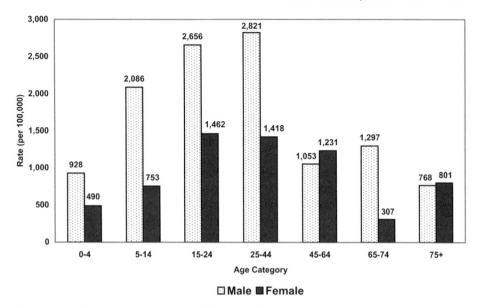

Figure 1.18 Incidence Rate (per 100,000) of Cut/Pierce Injuries

greatest differential occurring among those aged 5 to 14 years. For this age group, the rate among males was almost 3 times the rate among females. For those aged 45 years and older, the incidence rate of cut/pierce injury was greater among females, with the exception of persons aged 65 to 74 years, where the rate among males was nearly 4 times greater than that among females.

Figures 1.19 and 1.20 show the incidence rates of hospitalized and nonhospitalized cut/pierce injury, respectively. For hospitalized injuries, males had higher incidences than females for all age groups. Both males and females had their highest rates among people aged 15 to 24, at 67 and 26 per 100,000 persons, respectively. Females 45 to 64 and 75 years and older had higher rates of nonhospitalized cut/pierce injury compared to same-aged males. For all other age groups, males had higher rates of nonhospitalized cut/pierce injury.

Fire/Burns

In 2000, fires and burns resulted in 3,922 deaths, 24,519 hospitalized injuries, and more than 745,000 nonhospitalized injuries (see Table 1.2).

The highest rate of fire/burn injury among males occurred among the very young—those 0 to 4 years old (Figure 1.21). The rate of fire/burn injury among males 0 to 4 years old, 661 per 100,000, was more than 50% greater than the rate for 15-24 year-old males, who had the second highest rate (433 per 100,000) among males. The rate of fire/burn injury among females aged 45 to 64 was 512 per 100,000. This rate was 16% higher than the rate among females aged 0 to 4 (427 per 100,000) who had the second highest rate among females.

Those aged 75 years and older were at highest risk of death due to fires and burns, at 6.7 and 4.6 per 100,000 males and females, respectively (Figure 1.22). Males in

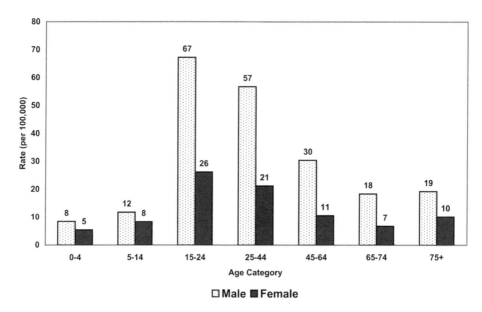

Figure 1.19 Incidence Rate (per 100,000) of Hospitalized Cut/Pierce Injuries

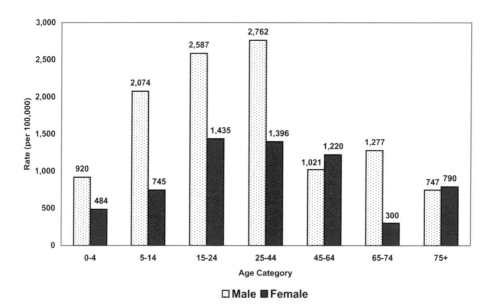

Figure 1.20 Incidence Rate (per 100,000) of Nonhospitalized Cut/Pierce Injuries

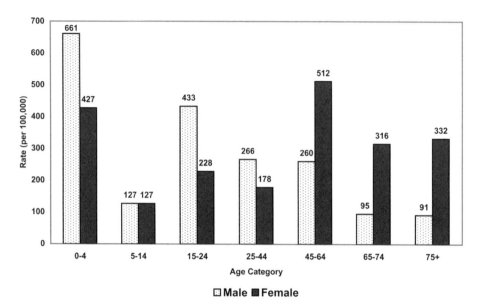

Figure 1.21 Incidence Rate (per 100,000) of Fire/Burn Injuries

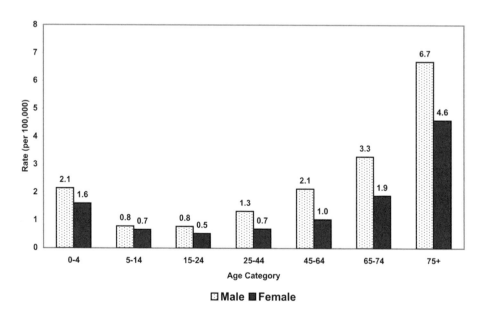

Figure 1.22 Incidence Rate (per 100,000) of Fatal Fire/Burn Injuries

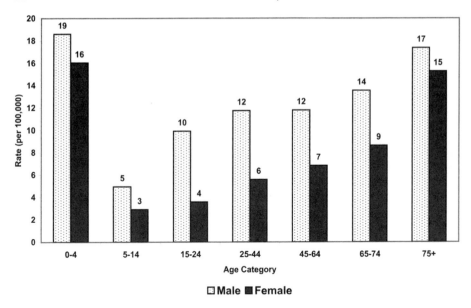

Figure 1.23 Incidence Rate (per 100,000) of Hospitalized Fire/Burn Injuries

every age category were more likely than females to die or be hospitalized from a fire or burn (Figures 1.22 and 1.23). The largest difference in burn hospitalizations was among those aged 15 to 24, where the rate for males was nearly 3 times the rate for females. For minor burns not requiring hospitalization (Figure 1.24), females 45 years and older were at consistently higher risk than males of the same age. The opposite is true for persons less than age 45 years, except for persons 5 to 14 years where the risk to males is slightly lower than the risks to females.

Residential fires are the leading cause of fire-related mortality. In 2003, residential fires accounted for 78% of fire-related injuries and 80% of fire-related deaths [Karter 2004]. In addition to older adults and young children, residential fires disproportionately affect African Americans, Native Americans, and the poorest Americans [U.S. Fire Administration 2001; Istre 2001].

Most victims of fires die from smoke or toxic gases and not from burns [Hall 2001]. Cooking is the primary cause of residential fires, and smoking is the leading cause of fire-related deaths [Ahrens 2001]. Alcohol use contributes to an estimated 40% of residential fire deaths [Smith 1999]. Smoke alarms decrease the chances of dying in a house fire by 40 to 50%. However, about one quarter of U.S. households lack working smoke alarms [Ahrens 2001].

Drowning/Submersion

Fatal drownings accounted for 4,168 deaths in 2000 (Table 1.2). There were 5,915 nonfatal drownings, of which 3,289 required hospitalization.

Drowning rates were markedly higher for persons less than 5 years old, nearly 4 times greater than any other age group (Figure 1.25). Figures 1.26 and 1.27 show the injury rates for fatal and hospitalized drowning injuries, respectively. Together, the

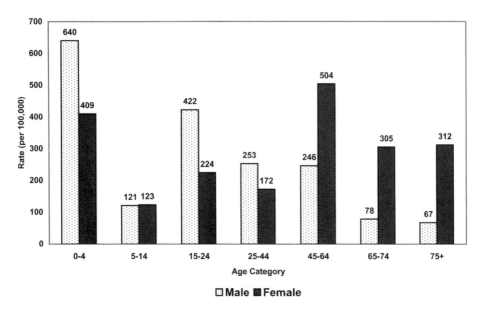

Figure 1.24 Incidence Rate (per 100,000) of Nonhospitalized Fire/Burn Injuries

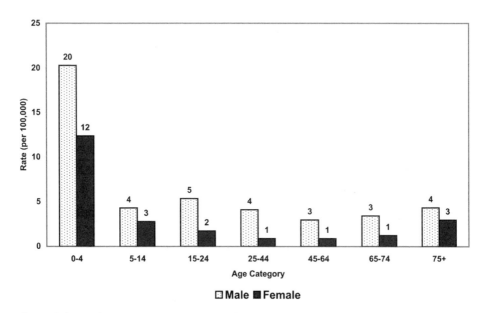

Figure 1.25 Incidence Rate (per 100,000) of Drowning/Submersion Injuries

27

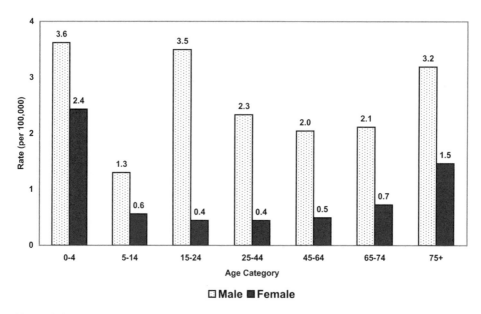

Figure 1.26 Incidence Rate (per 100,000) of Fatal Drowning/Submersion Injuries

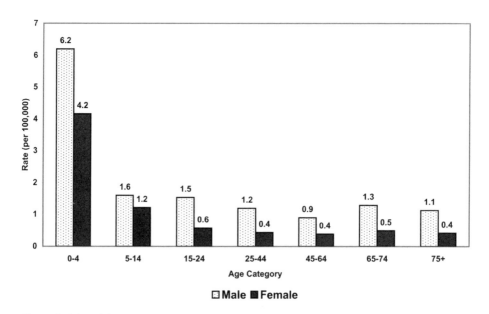

Figure 1.27 Incidence Rate (per 100,000) of Hospitalized Drowning/Submersion Injuries

figures demonstrate the importance of targeting prevention efforts at parents of very young children. The rates of fatal drownings were highest for both males and females 0 to 4 years old. For nonfatal hospitalized drowning injuries, the gap between the rates of 0- to 4-year-olds and others was much larger than for fatal injuries. For all age categories, the incidence of drowning was higher for males than for females. There were few nonfatal nonhospitalized drowning injuries for persons over 4 years old.

Where children are most likely to drown varies with age. Children under age 1 most often drown in bathtubs, buckets, or toilets [Brenner et al. 2001], while children aged 1 to 4 years most often drown in residential swimming pools [Brenner et al. 2001; Gilchrist et al. 2004]. As children get older, drownings more frequently occur in open water areas such as ponds, lakes, and rivers [Gilchrist et al. 2004]. Alcohol use is involved in about 25% to 50% of adolescent and adult deaths associated with water recreation [Howland et al. 1995; Howland & Hingson 1988]. Boating also carries risks for injuries, with drownings accounting for 70% of all boating fatalities [U.S. Coast Guard 2002].

Active, constant, visual supervision is the most effective way to prevent drownings and submersion injuries. Additional prevention strategies include the consistent use of personal floatation devices or life jackets, swimming in areas protected by lifeguards [Branche & Stewart 2001], water safety training, and measures to reduce children's access to unsupervised waters, such as the installation of 4-sided isolation fencing and self-latching gates around swimming pools and other hazards close to homes [Gilchrist et al. 2004; U.S. Consumer Product Safety Commission 1991].

Poisoning

In 2000, poisonings resulted in 20,261 deaths, 219,056 hospitalizations, and more than 1 million minor injuries (see Table 1.2).

Among males, the highest rates of poisoning injury were for those 0 to 4 years old, at 1,089 per 100,000 (Figure 1.28). Among females, the highest rate was for those 15 to 24 years old, at 1,309 per 100,000.

Nearly all deaths from poisoning occurred among persons over the age of 15 (Figure 1.29). Young adults aged 25 to 44 were at highest risk of a poisoning. Males aged 15 to 64 had a rate of poisoning death that is 2.3 times greater than the rate for females. The rates of hospitalized poisoning injury followed a similar pattern for age but not for gender (Figure 1.30). Persons aged 15 to 24 had the highest rate of hospitalized poisoning injury, followed by persons aged 25 to 44. For those aged 5 and older, rates of hospitalized poisoning injury among females were greater than among males, and among those 15 to 24, the rate was twice as high. No clear age/gender patterns emerge for risks of less serious poisoning not requiring hospitalization (Figure 1.31). Among males, those aged 0 to 4 had the highest rate (1,053 per 100,000 males), followed by those aged 65 to 74 (612 per 100,000 males). Among females, those aged 65 to 74 had the highest rate (1,182 per 100,000 females), closely followed by those aged 15 to 24 (1,153 per 100,000 females).

Progress has been made in reducing mortality among children from poisoning, especially by the use of childproof packaging. However, poisoning among adults, both fatal and nonfatal, is still a major—and growing—problem. Most fatal poisonings

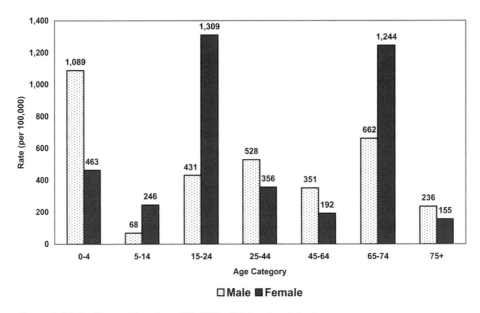

Figure 1.28 Incidence Rate (per 100,000) of Poisoning Injuries

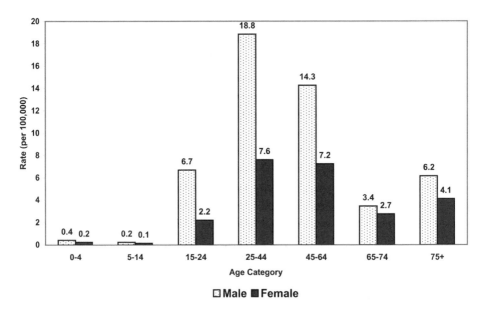

Figure 1.29 Incidence Rate (per 100,000) of Fatal Poisoning Injuries

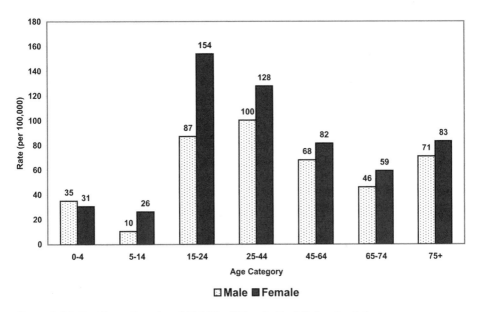

Figure 1.30 Incidence Rate (per 100,000) of Hospitalized Poisoning Injuries

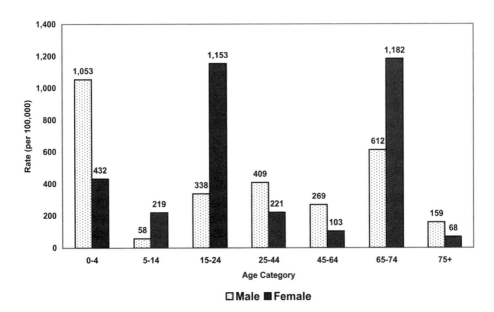

Figure 1.31 Incidence Rate (per 100,000) of Nonhospitalized Poisoning Injuries

among adults involve overdoses of 1 of 3 drugs: prescription narcotic painkillers, co-caine, or heroin [CDC MMWR 2004]. Strategies to reduce rates of misuse or abuse of these drugs are needed. Interdicting supplies of heroin and cocaine has proven diffi-cult. However, measures to reduce the volume of prescription narcotic painkillers being dispensed are promising strategies that should be tested.

Firearm/Gunshot

Firearm-/gunshot-related injuries totaled 131,013, of which 21% were fatal, 23% resulted in hospitalization and 55% were nonhospitalized (see Table 1.2). As shown in Appendix Table 1.11, 86% of all firearm injuries occurred among three age groups: 15 to 24 (32%), 25 to 44 (30%), and 5 to 14 (24%).

Figures 1.32 and 1.33 show the overall rate of firearm injuries and the rate of firearm fatalities, respectively, by age and gender. For both males and females, the highest rate of injury was for 15- to 24-year-olds; the rate of injury for males, 198 per 100,000, was 8 times the rate for females, 24 per 100,000. In fact, for all age groups, the rates of firearm-related injuries or fatalities were much larger for males than for females. For example, for persons, 75 years and older, the rate of death by firearm is over 15 times as large; as a result, approximately 89% (or 117,000) of firearm-related injuries were sustained by men. Among men, the rate of firearm-related fatalities was highest for those 75 years and older (36 per 100,000), followed by the rate for those between the ages of 15 and 24 years old (31 per 100,000) as shown in Figure 1.33.

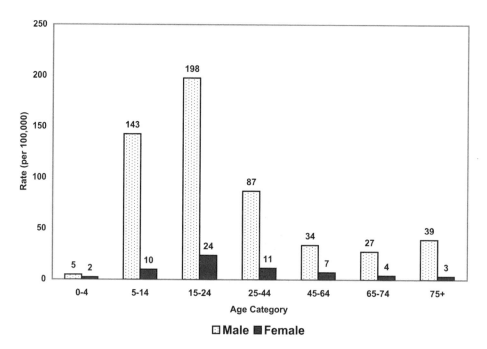

Figure 1.32 Incidence Rate (per 100,000) of Firearm/Gunshot Injuries

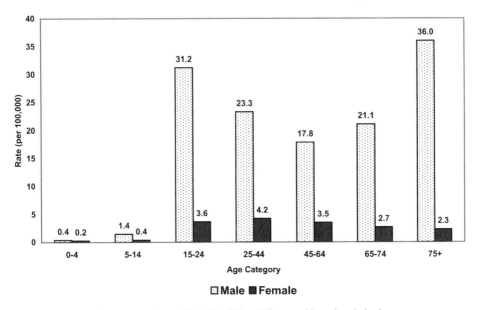

Figure 1.33 Incidence Rate (per 100,000) of Fatal Firearm/Gunshot Injuries

For firearm-related hospitalization, males aged 15 to 24 have the highest rate (63.2 per 100,000), which is more than 10 times the rate for females of the same age (Figure 1.34). For firearm-related injury that did not result in hospitalization, males aged 5 to 14 had the highest rate, which was 16 times that of females of the same age (Figure 1.35). It is likely that some of these nonhospitalized firearm injuries to young males may be due to BB guns or other kinds of less lethal firearms (which we could not separate from the firearm count because the necessary E-code detail often was missing). In contrast to firearm deaths, the elderly have comparatively lower rates of hospitalized and nonhospitalized firearm injuries.

Firearm injuries are an important public health problem in the United States contributing substantially each year to premature death, illness, and disability. Finding ways to prevent such injuries remains one of the most important challenges of public health. Some of the measures proposed to reduce the risk of a firearm-related death or injury are behavior oriented, including education around the safe storage and handling of guns, and school and community-based primary prevention programs [Hardy 2002; Grossman et al. 2000; Grossman et al. 2005]. Other measures (e.g., changing the design of firearms or personalizing them to make them more difficult to use unintentionally or intentionally if stolen or obtained illegally) are product-oriented [Teret et al. 2002]. There have also been legislative efforts (e.g., screening and licensing requirements for ownership, regulations for gun dealers, child access prevention laws, laws governing the transfer of firearms) to reduce the potential for firearm-related injury [Loftin et al. 1991; Lampert et al. 1998; Cummings et al. 1997; Eber et al. 2004]. Most of these measures, however, have not been adequately evaluated making it difficult to know which ones are the most effective in reducing firearm-related deaths or injuries [National Research Council 2005].

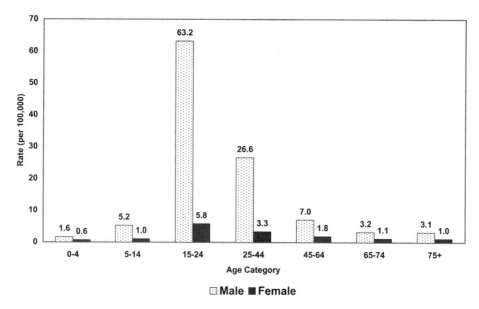

Figure 1.34 Incidence Rate (per 100,000) of Hospitalized Firearm/Gunshot Injuries

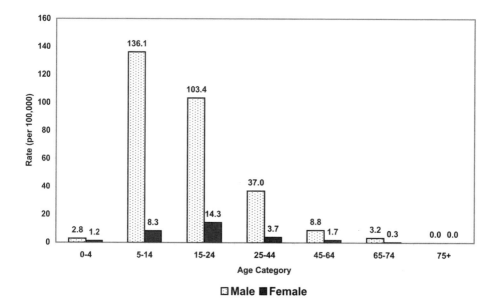

Figure 1.35 Incidence Rate (per 100,000) of Nonhospitalized Firearm/Gunshot Injuries

34

Incidence Data and Methods

The following sections present our approach to quantifying the incidence of injuries in 2000. To avoid double counting, we quantify injury incidence separately for the following categories:

1 Fatalities
2 Hospitalized injuries resulting in a live discharge
3 Nonhospitalized nonfatal injuries, which result in:
   a. a hospital emergency department (ED) visit but no overnight admission
   b. an office-based medical visit but no hospital admission or ED visit
   c. a hospital outpatient visit but no other hospital or office-based treatment
   d. medical treatment, for example by a dentist or a chiropractor, but no hospital-based or medical office treatment

If an injured patient is treated in multiple settings the incident is classified based on the hierarchy above, which roughly denotes injury severity. For example, if an injured patient presents at the ED and is later admitted to the hospital and subsequently seen in a physician's office, that patient would be included in the incidence count for injuries requiring a hospitalization (no. 2 in the list above). If another injured patient were seen in the ED and is subsequently seen in a physician's office, but never admitted to the hospital, she would be counted in the incidence count for injuries requiring an ED visit (no. 3a in the list above). This strategy allows for summing injuries across settings to uniquely quantify the total incidence of injuries for the population. Separate data sources were used to estimate the incidence of injuries for 1 through 3 above. The data sources and methods are described in the following sections and outlined in Table 1.5.

Fatalities

Fatal injury counts came from 2000 National Vital Statistics System (NVSS) data, which includes a census of fatalities in the United States. NVSS data are compiled by the states from medical examiner and coroner records, and pooled by the National Center for Health Statistics (NCHS). These data provide information on (among other variables) the age, sex, race, and county and state of residence of the deceased; cause of death is coded to the 10th revision of the International Classification of Diseases (ICD-10). Injuries are identified using the following underlying cause of death mechanisms: motor vehicle/other road user, falls, struck by/against, cut/pierce, fire/burn, poisoning, drowning/submersion, firearm/gunshot, or other. Some mechanisms (e.g., machinery incidents) are included in total counts but are not discussed in detail in this book. We collapsed the detailed external cause codes into the mechanism categories recommended by the International Collaborative Effort (ICE) on Injury Statistics, using rules posted on the ICE page of the NCHS web site,[2] then further collapsed them into the mechanism groupings reported in this book.

---

[2] Cause codes in ICD-10, like E codes in ICD-9, embody information on both injury mechanism and intent. The matrix for categorizing ICD-10 cause codes into mechanism and intent groupings, developed by NCHS, can be found at http://www.cdc.gov/nchs/data/ice/icd10_transcode.pdf.

Table 1.5 Data Sources for Estimating Incidence of Injuries, 2000

Injury Category	Main Source	Adjustments Using Other Data
Fatal	2000 NVSS—a census of fatalities in the United States	2000 FARS was used to categorize injuries by mechanism for motor-vehicle occupant, motorcyclist, pedestrian, and pedalcyclist deaths in motor-vehicle crashes on public roads
Nonfatal injuries requiring hospitalization	2000 HCUP-NIS—a nationally representative cluster sample of discharges from nonfederal, short-term, general, and other specialty hospitals, excluding hospital units of institutions	Pooled 1997–98 hospital discharge census data for Maryland, Vermont, and New Jersey provided readmission rates by diagnosis group that were used to remove readmissions (average readmisison rate 6.3%)
	Mechanism was missing for 17% of cases. This information was inferred from cases with known information and the same diagnosis, age group, and sex	1999 National Nursing Home Survey (NNHS) data was used to reduce counts by the number of injured patients who were transferred to and subsequently died in a nursing home (5,226)
Nonfatal injuries not requiring hospitalization		
Injuries requiring an emergency department visit	2001 NEISS–AIP—a nationally representative sample of Emergency Department discharges for injury	1999–2000 NHAMCS-ED data was used to construct the distribution of injuries by diagnosis group and severity
Injuries requiring only an office-based visit and/or a hospital outpatient visit	1999–2000 NHAMCS-OPD and NAMCS—nationally representative surveys of hospital outpatient department and ambulatory medical care visits, respectively	Totals were adjusted to match the corresponding counts of injury patients (as opposed to visits) treated only in doctors' offices and only in outpatient departments from 1999 MEPS

The National Center for Health Statistics categorized all 1,200 ICD-10 injury diagnosis codes into the body region, body part, and nature of injury categories with the aim of trying to be as compatible as possible with the Barell Injury Diagnosis Matrix (www.cdc.gov/nchs/about/otheract/ice/barellmatrix.htm), which is widely used to classify nonfatal injuries. This was made more difficult because of the additional diagnosis codes (referred to as "S" and "T" codes in ICD-10) and because the axis of definition for the diagnosis codes changed between ICD-9 and ICD-10. While death certificates for injury are supposed to list all injury diagnoses involved in the death, there is no formal guidance on how to identify a principal injury diagnosis. Until such guidance is formalized by the World Health Organization's (WHO) Mortality Reference Group, we assumed that each listed injury diagnosis contributed equally to the death. For example, if a death certificate listed a spinal cord injury (SCI) and a traumatic brain injury (TBI), our tables would include one half death due to SCI and one half death due to TBI. Other assumptions are possible.

A drawback of NVSS data is that medical examiners and coroners often do not record whether an occupant killed in a motor-vehicle crash is a driver or passenger.

In the 2000 NVSS data, 35% of motor vehicle traffic deaths fell into the category "Motor vehicle, other unspecified," typically because their seating position was unknown. However, the National Highway Traffic Safety Administration (NHTSA) has developed its own motor vehicle crash mortality census, the Fatality Analysis Reporting System (FARS), which we used to get more accurate categorizations. We used the 2000 FARS census of motor-vehicle fatalities to get percentages for motor-vehicle-occupant, motorcyclist, pedestrian, and pedalcyclist deaths in motor-vehicle crashes on public roads within 30 days of any crash reported in the NVSS data; using the FARS data, we were able to assign specific categories to 41,828 of the 42,348 NVSS fatalities. Fatalities that did not occur on public roads (e.g., of children run over in driveways, dirt-bike racers, dune buggy drivers) remain in the unspecified category if the death certificate placed them there. This procedure reduced the deaths with role unspecified to 1% of the total.

Hospitalized Injuries Resulting in a Live Discharge

We used the 2000 Healthcare Cost and Utilization Project–Nationwide Inpatient Sample (HCUP-NIS) to develop incidence-based estimates of the number of injuries resulting in hospitalizations with live discharges in 2000. The HCUP-NIS provides information annually on approximately 5 to 8 million inpatient stays (that resulted in live discharges in 2000) from about 1,000 hospitals. These hospitals represent a 20% sample of nonfederal, short-term, general, and other specialty hospitals, excluding hospital units of institutions, drawn from a convenience sample of 33 states that have hospital discharge census data. All discharges from sampled hospitals are included in the HCUP-NIS database, and sampling weights are included to allow for generating national estimates.

Two accounting issues arise with these data. First, some HCUP-NIS discharges recorded in 2000 would result from injury events that occurred prior to 2000; however, roughly the same number of patients are excluded from the 2000 sample because they were not discharged by the end of the year. Therefore, this database is expected to accurately quantify hospitalized injury incidence for 2000. Second, to avoid double-counting individuals who were discharged and then subsequently died in a nursing home, we subtracted the 5,226 injury deaths in nursing homes in 2000 from the hospitalized survivor count, since an inpatient stay with live discharge likely preceded a nursing home stay that ended in injury-related death. Individuals with a live discharge who subsequently died outside a medical facility (i.e., hospital, nursing home) will be double counted as fatal injuries and hospitalized injuries; however, we expect this number to be extremely small.

Each HCUP-NIS record contains patient-level utilization and resource-use information included in a typical discharge abstract, including ICD-9-CM diagnosis codes. We included all records that indicate a live discharge and an injury diagnosis in any of the first three diagnosis fields, based on recommendations of an expert panel.[3]

---

[3]Since the HCUP-NIS comprises hospital discharge data published by the various participating states, each record is subject to the data limitations of the state and the hospital that it came from. The number of diagnosis slots available for a given case is typically 9 or 10, but it can vary from 6 to 25.

Nonfatal injuries are identified by ICD-9-CM diagnosis codes recommended by the ICE injury working group and the STIPDA, as outlined at the beginning of this chapter. These criteria resulted in an analytical file of 343,764 hospitalized injury records. One shortcoming of these data is that they do not differentiate between initial admissions and readmissions. Therefore, because some of these cases might be rehospitalizations for the same injury, we adjusted the incidence estimates downward using readmission probabilities based on diagnosis groups and age. We estimated these probabilities from over 200,000 hospital admissions in pooled 1997–98 discharge census data for Maryland, Vermont, and New Jersey, three states that flag readmissions. Although these states might not be representative of national readmission rates, their discharge records are the only available recent and reliable source of population-based information on the readmission rates for specific injury diagnoses.

Using these data, we estimated readmission probabilities for select diagnosis groups based on the Barell Injury Diagnosis Matrix stratified by age groups. The percentage of injury admissions that are readmissions ranged from barely above 0% to nearly 15%, with an average of 6.3%. By comparison, the percentage that are readmissions in the 1997–99 Medical Expenditure Panel Survey (MEPS) is 8.7% (unweighted), with annual estimates ranging from 7.9% to 9.6%. Although the MEPS estimates are slightly larger, they may include some cases where the readmission is actually a transfer between services (e.g., acute care and rehabilitation) in one hospital.

Classification by Mechanism

Our mechanism classifications were limited by the fact that, in states where discharge records do not use a separate field for E (external cause: mechanism and intent) codes, patients with multiple injuries or diagnoses (e.g., the elderly) are less likely to be assigned E codes due to limitations in the number of diagnosis/E-code fields. As a result, in only 87% of cases could the mechanism of injury be identified either by a diagnosis (for drownings, poisonings, and burns) or by an external (E) code (all E codes except 849, 869.4, 870–879 or 930–949, for motor vehicles, falls, firearms, etc.).

For cases where no E code was present in the hospital record, we imputed E codes based on the distribution of E-coded cases with the same primary diagnosis, age group, (0–4, 5–14, 15–24, 25–44, 45–64, 65–74, 75+) and sex. For example, if all of the E-coded cases for a particular diagnosis, age, and gender group were split equally (after weighting) between two E codes, then we randomly assigned these E codes to the noncoded cases in the same strata ensuring that 50% of the (weighted) noncoded cases were assigned each code. Using this approach, we were able to assign E codes to all but 0.33% of cases. For the remaining cases, we imputed the E codes based on all cases with the same diagnosis, no matter the age and sex.

By diagnosis, the percentage not E coded ranged from 0% for vertebral column fractures without spinal cord injuries and crushing injuries of the face and of multiple body regions to a high of 50% for poisonings by bacterial vaccines, 53% for jaw dislocations, and 61% for injuries from radiation. Of 179 diagnosis groups (at the three digit ICD level), another 13, including 6 for nerve injuries and 3 for multiple or nonspecific fractures, were missing E codes for more than 30% of cases. The 17 diagnosis groups with large (>30%) missing E codes comprise less than 1.5% of the injury discharges.

Classification by Body Part and Nature of Injury

Based on the principal diagnosis, all injured persons discharged from the hospital are classified into one of 183 injury categories defined by body part and nature of injury. In assigning these categories, we used the Barell Injury Diagnosis Matrix, which maps ICD-9-CM codes into 36 body parts and 12 natures of injury. We broke out poisonings and foreign bodies as separate categories, removing them from the "system wide and late effects" category in the Barell matrix.

Classification by Body Region and Severity

All injured persons discharged from the hospital are classified into one of the 72 injury categories defined by body region and severity of the most severe injury sustained. Body region and injury severity were determined using ICDMAP-90 [Johns Hopkins University and Tri-Analytics, Inc., 1997], a program that estimates Abbreviated Injury Score (AIS) [Association for the Advancement of Automotive Medicine, 1990] from the patient's age and ICD-9-CM injury diagnoses. AIS describe the severity of injury on a scale of 1 (minor threat to life) to 6 (virtually unsurvivable) for each of nine body regions. The maximum AIS is the greatest of the AIS scores of the patients multiple injuries, and the principal AIS body region is the body region that sustained the injury with the greatest severity. AIS are not available for poisoning, drowning, suffocation, or codes added to ICD-9-CM after 1996 when ICDMAP was completed. In multiple-injury cases where two injuries were of the same severity, we selected the principal injury as the classifying injury.

ICDMAP was able to assign AIS threat-to-life scores (other than unknown) to 97% of hospital-admitted survivors (excluding poisonings, suffocations, and drownings), but only 91% of nonadmitted survivors because nonadmitted diagnoses were less specific. ICDMAP also codes conservatively, meaning severity sometimes is understated.

Nonhospitalized Injuries

Injuries Requiring an Emergency Department Visit

We estimated injuries treated in the emergency department (ED) from the 2001 National Electronic Injury Surveillance System–All Injury Program (NEISS-AIP), which collects data from EDs at 66 hospitals, supplemented by the 1999–2000 National Hospital Ambulatory Medical Care Survey (NHAMCS), which surveys approximately 500 hospitals. We used NEISS-AIP (2001 is the first complete year of

NEISS data collection) to generate numerical estimates of injuries and NHAMCS to construct a more detailed distribution by diagnosis group.

The NEISS-AIP data include information on first visits associated with injuries not resulting in fatalities (i.e., any follow-up ED visits for the same injury are excluded). These data used the Consumer Product Safety Commission's (CPSC) definition of injury, which includes not only all of the diagnoses we classify as injury but also dermatitis and conjunctivitis. We dropped 2,237 patients whose diagnosis was dermatitis or conjunctivitis. To avoid double counting, we further excluded patients who were subsequently admitted to the hospital or transferred to another hospital (27,357 unweighted cases or 5.7%). We also excluded those few cases for which the patient's disposition (337 cases), age (135 cases), or sex (87 cases) was missing. This left data on 451,859 (unweighted) injury survivors who were treated in the ED and released (not admitted to the hospital) during 2001.

The NEISS-AIP data and NHAMCS data differ in several ways. First, NEISS-AIP codes major external cause groupings based on ICD-9 guidelines; NHAMCS codes using ICD-9-CM E codes. Second, NEISS-AIP focuses on the precipitating cause of injury, the first in the chain of events that led to the injury, rather than the direct cause of injury. For example, an unintentional fall into a stove that led to a burn injury would be classified as an unintentional fall in NEISS-AIP. In many cases, the precipitating and immediate causes are the same, but in some cases, primarily cases coded as falls or struck by/against, they are not. Third, NEISS-AIP only collects data on one body part and, unlike NHAMCS, only one diagnosis, which the attending physician determines is the patient's principal injury diagnosis. The NEISS-AIP diagnosis classification system consists of 26 body parts and 31 injury codes; these are almost entirely matched according to mechanism to the ICD-9-CM-based Barell matrix. Table 1.6 details the matrix categories that had to be collapsed in this book in order to match the NEISS-AIP data fully.

As stated above, we used NEISS-AIP to generate numerical estimates of injuries, and NHAMCS to construct a more detailed distribution by mechanism. NHAMCS is better for capturing mechanism because the data entered into NHAMCS come directly from hospital staff and Census Bureau field representatives who code the verbatim text of the mechanism of injury and include up to 3 ICD-9-CM injury mechanisms for each record. For the years 1999 and 2000 combined, the total unweighted NHAMCS cases of ED-treated injuries not admitted to the hospital or resulting in a fatality was 12,718. The weighted case count (including cases lacking E codes) differed from the NEISS count by only 2.5%.

We used the NEISS estimates as the primary estimates both because the much larger NEISS sample size supports more detailed tabular breakdowns and because a larger percentage of NHAMCS cases are missing information on mechanism (15% versus 3%). However, we used detailed diagnosis coding in NHAMCS to fill out diagnosis information in the NEISS estimates. To do this, we multiplied the NHAMCS case weights by the ratio of the NEISS total injury count to the NHAMCS total injury count. We used the resulting estimates to analyze the distribution of injuries by diagnosis group classified using the ICD-9-CM-based Barell matrix and to AIS-score the injuries.

Table 1.6 Conversion of Selected Categories from ICD-9-CM to NEISS

ICD-9-CM Matrix of Mechanism of Injury	NEISS Matrix of Mechanism of Injury
"Fire/flame" and "hot object/substance"	"Fire/burn"
"Motor vehicle traffic pedestrian" and "other pedestrian"	"Pedestrian"
"Motor vehicle traffic pedalcyclist" and "other pedalcyclist"	"Pedalcyclist"

Classification by Mechanism

Using the NEISS-AIP, we grouped E codes into mechanism categories using the modified morbidity version of the ICD-9 Framework for Presenting Injury Mortality Data developed by ICE, which uses the more detailed codes from the U.S. clinical modification, found at http://www.cdc.gov/ncipc/whatsnew/matrix2.htm. Differences between the ICE matrix and classification schemes employed by NEISS-AIP, which was used to estimate the incidence of ED treated injuries, necessitated the collapsing of a few mechanism categories for the sake of consistency (Table 1.6).

Injuries Requiring an Office-Based Visit and/or Outpatient Visit

We estimated the number of injuries resulting in medical treatment without hospitalization or ED treatment from the 1999 to 2000 National Ambulatory Medical Care Survey (NAMCS), the 1999 to 2000 NHAMCS hospital outpatient department sample, and the 1999 Medical Expenditure Panel Survey (MEPS). The NAMCS is a national survey designed to provide reliable information about the provision and use of ambulatory medical care services in the United States. These data were based on a sample of visits to nonfederally employed, office-based (or freestanding clinic-based) physicians and osteopaths who principally engage in direct patient care. Data are collected from physicians, with coding and quality control procedures paralleling the NHAMCS data. They include up to three ICD-9-CM diagnoses for each case.

We estimated the incidence of injury visits treated only in doctors' offices by pooling 1999 and 2000 NAMCS data and estimating yearly averages. Similarly, our estimate of outpatient clinic visits relied on 1999 and 2000 NHAMCS data. To be consistent with the inpatient analysis, we limited our selection to those visits coded by NAMCS or NHAMCS as an acute case of injury or poisoning. To avoid double counting, we excluded NAMCS cases where the patient was admitted to an ED or hospital, or returned to a referring physician. For the years 1999 and 2000 combined, there were 1,885 doctor's office cases (unweighted) and 2,804 outpatient department cases (unweighted).

The NAMCS/NHAMCS data cannot be used to estimate incidence directly because they count injury visits, as opposed to injuries. They do indicate if a patient was treated previously by another physician or was admitted to a hospital following the visit, but they do not distinguish other acute-care follow-up visits from initial visits and do not always indicate whether patients were treated in other settings. To arrive at a unique injury incidence count for cases treated only in doctors' offices, we adjusted the NAMCS and NHAMCS outpatient department totals to match the corresponding count of injuries (not visits) treated only in doctors' offices and only in outpatient departments from the 1999 MEPS.

MEPS is a nationally representative survey of the civilian noninstitutionalized population that quantifies individuals' use of health services and corresponding medical expenditures. MEPS contains a unique record for each medical condition self-reported by participants during the year. These self-reported conditions are classified by trained medical coders based on 3-digit ICD-9 diagnosis codes. A unique condition identifier links medical conditions to medical treatment at the following locations: inpatient, emergency department, outpatient, office-based, dental, and home health. These data allow us to identify individuals who sustained injuries, stratified by treatment location. As with administrative claims data, more than one ICD code may be associated with each record. So we assumed that the first-listed code, which is the first condition self-reported by the MEPS participant, represents the primary diagnosis.

Since MEPS tracks medical care at the individual level, it allows for identifying the number of visits in each treatment location associated with a given injury. Table 1.7 shows that roughly 4 physician office visits result for injuries initially treated in this setting, and slightly less than 3 visits result, on average, for injuries initially treated in a hospital outpatient department. Moreover, as the MEPS data show, many injury patients have more than one injury in a year—as shown by the difference between rows 3 and 2. We use the MEPS unique injury counts of those who sustain a nonfatal nonadmitted injury to ensure that no double counting occurs for injuries resulting in multiple visits or treated in multiple settings. MEPS estimates a total of 19.6 million unique injuries treated in doctor's offices (without an ED visit or inpatient stay), and 0.6 million treated in an outpatient department (without an ED visit, inpatient stay, or doctor's office visit).

To allow for stratifying injuries by mechanism, information not available in MEPS, we reduced the NAMCS and NHAMCS visit counts to match the MEPS injury counts within each age category (0–4, 5–14, 15–24, 25–44, 45–64, 65–74, 75+) and gender strata. To arrive at these counts, we first removed NAMCS and NHAMCS cases within each strata that lacked E codes or whose E code was coded as "unspecified" (approximately 19% of cases from each file). Within the 7 broad mechanism categories in MEPS (motor vehicle, fall, firearm, other weapon, fire/burn, poisoning, drowning, and other), we then proportionately reduced the weights

Table 1.7 Estimates of Injuries and Injury Outpatient Visits Using MEPS and NAMCS/NHAMCS

| | Doctor's Office | | Hospital Outpatient Department | |
	NAMCS	MEPS	NHAMCS	MEPS
Total injury visits	88,369,000	98,855,000	9,417,000	8,717,000
Total injury patients	33,249,000*	25,244,000	4,283,000*	3,234,000
Injury patients not treated in EDs or as inpatients		19,589,000		591,000 (Not treated in doctor's office, or clinic)

* Double-counts some patients with multiple visits.

of all remaining visits within each strata until the weighted NAMCS and NHAMCS counts matched the MEPS counts for office-based and outpatient injuries, respectively (i.e., we multiplied the weights times the ratio of the MEPS count to the NAMCS or NHAMCS count). This approach may make the estimates by mechanism less reliable than estimates from the other data sets, but it preserves the accuracy of the total count with respect to treatment location.

Classification by Mechanism

NAMCS and NHAMCS use E codes, thus allowing the data to be classified by mechanism as described in the inpatient analyses. Mechanism codes are also included on the NEISS data. MEPS records only 7 broad mechanism categories, which forces us to collapse tables that included MEPS incidence data into these broad categories (i.e., motor vehicle, fall, firearm, other weapon, fire/burn, poisoning, drowning, other). For this reason, our tables exclude 2 million oro-facial injury patients annually (captured in MEPS) who were treated only in dental offices.

Classification by Body Part and Nature of Injury

NAMCS and NHAMCS use ICD-9-CM diagnosis codes, allowing the data to be collapsed into the Barell matrix's body part and nature of injury categories in the same manner as hospital-admitted injuries. The NHAMCS-ED sample rather than the NEISS data are used in the Barell matrix tables. We also ran ICDMAP90 on these cases to estimate AIS scores.

Denominators for Rate Calculations

To compute rates, we used population counts from the same 1999 MEPS data that provided most of the injury incidence counts. These data cover the civilian, noninstitutionalized resident population of the United States. Its 276.4 million estimate (Table 1.8) is only slightly lower than the Census Bureau's broader estimates of 279.0

Table 1.8 Civilian Noninstitutionalized Resident Population by Age and Sex, United States, 1999

Age Group	Male	Female	Total
Total	*134,603,000*	*141,807,000*	*276,410,000*
0–4	10,270,000	9,416,000	19,686,000
5–14	20,940,000	20,340,000	41,280,000
15–24	18,980,000	18,390,000	37,370,000
25–44	40,320,000	42,330,000	82,650,000
45–64	28,910,000	30,850,000	59,760,000
65–74	7,989,000	9,653,000	17,642,000
75+	5,924,000	9,219,000	15,143,000
Missing	1,270,000	1,609,000	2,879,000

Source: 1999 Medical Expenditure Panel Study.

million total U.S. residents, including those in institutions, for 1999 and 281.4 million for 2000 [U.S. Census Bureau 2003].

Limitations of Incidence Estimates

This chapter provides up-to-date and comprehensive estimates of the incidence of injuries in the United States. The estimates are gleaned from myriad data sources; as such, all limitations inherent to these data can be applied to the current analysis. These include issues associated with sample selection, data reliability, and precision. For example, MEPS is limited to the civilian noninstitutionalized population, and therefore our estimates for injuries treated in outpatient settings (which is based on MEPS counts) may be biased downward. Other data sets did not contain complete coding information and thus required the use of algorithms to impute missing data. This not only increases the lack of precision around the estimates, but may result in additional bias. Regrettably, due to a lack of detail on mechanism of injury, we were forced to drop nearly 2 million oro-facial injuries treated in dental offices. Injuries treated by chiropractors, acupuncturists, and other alternative medicine healers are also likely to be excluded, as are injuries that, although potentially severe, did not receive medical attention. Regardless, the results presented above represent the best available estimates of injury incidence in the United States today. Future studies will improve upon the methodology and results.

Appendix 1.1 Incidence Counts and Rates (per 100,000) of Injuries by Nature of Injury, 2000

Nature	Fatal		Hospitalized		Nonhospitalized		Total	
	Incidence	Rate	Incidence	Rate	Incidence	Rate	Incidence	Rate
Total	*149,075*	*54*	*1,869,857*	*676*	*48,108,166*	*17,405*	*50,127,098*	*18,135*
Fracture	12,158	4	920,520	333	6,082,003	2,200	7,014,681	2,538
Dislocation	213	0	22,298	8	1,351,865	489	1,374,376	497
Sprain/strain	15	0	80,037	29	14,921,730	5,398	15,001,782	5,427
Internal organ	12,248	4	187,116	68	400,044	145	599,408	217
Open wound	27,959	10	155,238	56	8,741,130	3,162	8,924,327	3,229
Amputation	106	0	7,641	3	65,922	24	73,669	27
Blood vessel	2,089	1	5,910	2	14,735	5	22,734	8
Superficial/contusion	284	0	136,675	49	10,331,651	3,738	10,468,611	3,787
Crushing	730	0	3,086	1	182,850	66	186,665	68
Burn	1,043	0	26,616	10	763,834	276	791,492	286
Nerve	47	0	4,786	2	99,936	36	104,769	38
Unspecified	53,097	19	40,804	15	2,525,998	914	2,619,899	948
System-wide	39,085	14	279,131	101	2,626,469	950	2,944,686	1,065

Appendix 1.2 Incidence Counts and Rates (per 100,000) of Injuries by Body Part, 2000

Body Part	Fatal		Hospitalized		Nonhospitalized		Total	
	Incidence	Rate	Incidence	Rate	Incidence	Rate	Incidence	Rate
Total	*149,075*	*54*	*1,869,857*	*676*	*48,108,166*	*17,405*	*50,127,098*	*18,135*
TBI type 1	40,148	15	106,436	39	875,896	317	1,022,480	370
TBI type 2	0	0	43,668	16	271,590	98	315,258	114
TBI type 3	0	0	5,483	2	0	0	5,483	2
Other head	726	0	19,281	7	745,111	270	765,118	277
Face	40	0	67,719	24	2,177,829	788	2,245,588	812
Eye	24	0	15,246	6	1,324,594	479	1,339,865	485
Neck	3,786	1	3,816	1	67,216	24	74,818	27
Head/face/neck unspec	26	0	38,023	14	2,077,065	751	2,115,114	765
SCI cervical	163	0	5,491	2	4,406	2	10,060	4
SCI thoracic/dorsal	3	0	2,483	1	6,338	2	8,825	3
SCI lumbar	0	0	1,502	1	0	0	1,502	1
SCI sacrum/coccyx	0	0	107	0	0	0	107	0
SCI unspec vertebra	594	0	732	0	5,242	2	6,568	2
VCI cervical	448	0	20,869	8	2,379,552	861	2,400,869	869
VCI thoracic/dorsal	14	0	20,136	7	582,606	211	602,757	218
VCI lumbar	76	0	39,634	14	1,601,523	579	1,641,233	594
VCI sacrum/coccyx	0	0	4,127	1	29,034	11	33,161	12
VCI unspec vertebra	229	0	1,451	1	26,112	9	27,792	10
Chest	12,262	4	101,008	37	1,019,545	369	1,132,815	410
Abdomen	2,080	1	51,828	19	110,910	40	164,818	60
Pelvis/urogenital	147	0	68,898	25	1,399,323	506	1,468,367	531
Trunk	8,109	3	12,130	4	288,798	104	309,036	112
Back/buttock	526	0	10,787	4	1,068,953	387	1,080,266	391
Shoulder/upper arm	350	0	110,150	40	2,823,794	1,022	2,934,293	1,062
Forearm/elbow	73	0	77,421	28	1,946,786	704	2,024,280	732
Hand/wrist/fingers	198	0	71,441	26	7,524,182	2,722	7,595,821	2,748
Other/unspec upper limb	264	0	16,292	6	752,606	272	769,163	278
Hip	5,417	2	294,374	106	405,475	147	705,267	255
Upper leg/thigh	895	0	54,811	20	170,209	62	225,914	82
Knee	156	0	35,615	13	1,640,688	594	1,676,459	607
Lower leg/ankle	514	0	182,465	66	3,161,451	1,144	3,344,430	1,210
Foot/toes	13	0	42,848	16	2,418,570	875	2,461,431	891
Other/unspec lower limb	345	0	46,088	17	2,787,559	1,008	2,833,991	1,025
Other/multiple/NEC	18,049	7	1,149	0	1,530	1	20,728	7
Unspecified	14,316	5	17,216	6	5,787,206	2,094	5,818,738	2,105
System-wide	39,085	14	279,131	101	2,626,469	950	2,944,686	1,065

Appendix 1.3 Incidence Counts and Rates (per 100,000) of Injuries by Detailed Mechanism and Gender, 2000

Injury Mechanism	Fatal Incidence	Fatal Rate	Hospitalized Incidence	Hospitalized Rate	Nonhospitalized Incidence	Nonhospitalized Rate	Total Incidence	Total Rate
Total	*149,075*	*54*	*1,869,857*	*676*	*48,108,166*	*17,405*	*50,127,098*	*18,135*
MV occupant	33,448	12	182,634	66	3,194,119	1,156	3,410,201	1,234
Motorcyclist	2,862	1	22,957	8	230,683	83	256,502	93
Pedalcyclist	866	0	25,063	9	613,563	222	639,492	231
Pedestrian	6,106	2	30,128	11	168,133	61	204,367	74
MVT unspecified	520	0	15,400	6	483,956	175	499,876	181
Other transport	3,114	1	41,235	15	1,105,042	400	1,149,391	416
Fall	14,052	5	854,589	309	10,698,101	3,870	11,566,742	4,185
Struck by/against	1,301	0	85,687	31	10,587,192	3,830	10,674,180	3,862
Machinery	679	0	15,756	6	595,416	215	611,851	221
Firearm/gunshot	28,722	10	29,609	11	72,682	26	131,013	47
Cut/pierce	2,293	1	71,129	26	4,050,663	1,465	4,124,085	1,492
Poisoning	20,261	7	219,056	79	1,028,148	372	1,267,465	459
Fire/burn	3,922	1	24,519	9	745,935	270	774,376	280
Inhalation/suffocation	12,131	4	10,169	4	158,160	57	180,460	65
Drown/submersion	4,168	2	3,289	1	2,626	1	10,083	4
Bite/sting	0	0	27,126	10	3,301,086	1,194	3,328,345	1,204
Natural/environmental	1,756	1	15,265	6	848,422	307	865,310	313
Overexertion	13	0	42,462	15	5,187,412	1,877	5,229,887	1,892
Other specified	1,984	1	64,335	23	4,232,277	1,531	4,298,596	1,555
Unspecified	10,877	4	89,448	32	804,551	291	904,876	327
Male	*103,900*	*77*	*901,798*	*670*	*25,559,533*	*18,989*	*26,565,232*	*19,736*
MV occupant	21,944	16	100,110	74	1,411,154	1,048	1,533,207	1,139
Motorcyclist	2,589	2	20,370	15	209,015	155	231,974	172
Pedalcyclist	752	1	19,803	15	446,156	331	466,712	347
Pedestrian	4,264	3	19,008	14	82,838	62	106,110	79
MVT unspecified	137	0	8,603	6	204,588	152	213,328	158
Other transport	2,559	2	27,996	21	658,226	489	688,781	512
Fall	7,647	6	306,583	228	4,887,446	3,631	5,201,676	3,865
Struck by/against	1,109	1	66,833	50	6,592,359	4,898	6,660,301	4,948
Machinery	651	0	14,214	11	472,902	351	487,767	362
Firearm/gunshot	24,638	18	26,278	20	66,113	49	117,029	87
Cut/pierce	1,678	1	50,354	37	2,550,052	1,895	2,602,084	1,933
Poisoning	13,721	10	90,090	67	485,089	360	588,900	438
Fire/burn	2,333	2	15,069	11	354,586	263	371,988	276
Inhalation/suffocation	8,140	6	5,464	4	125,979	94	139,583	104
Drown/submersion	3,198	2	2,166	2	1,652	1	7,016	5
Bite/sting	0	0	13,877	10	1,347,012	1,001	1,360,979	1,011
Natural/environmental	1,136	1	9,279	7	208,986	155	219,311	163
Overexertion	10	0	22,576	17	3,064,784	2,277	3,087,370	2,294
Other specified	1,582	1	38,018	28	1,872,924	1,391	1,912,524	1,421
Unspecified	5,812	4	45,108	34	517,673	385	568,593	422

Injury Mechanism	Fatal		Hospitalized		Nonhospitalized		Total	
	Incidence	Rate	Incidence	Rate	Incidence	Rate	Incidence	Rate
Female	*45,175*	*32*	*968,059*	*683*	*22,548,634*	*15,902*	*23,561,868*	*16,616*
MV occupant	11,504	8	82,525	58	1,782,965	1,257	1,876,994	1,324
Motorcyclist	273	0	2,587	2	21,668	15	24,528	17
Pedal cyclist	114	0	5,260	4	167,407	118	172,781	122
Pedestrian	1,842	1	11,120	8	85,295	60	98,257	69
MVT unspecified	383	0	6,797	5	279,368	197	286,548	202
Other transport	555	0	13,240	9	446,816	315	460,611	325
Fall	6,405	5	548,006	386	5,810,655	4,098	6,365,066	4,489
Struck by/against	192	0	18,855	13	3,994,833	2,817	4,013,880	2,831
Machinery	28	0	1,542	1	122,514	86	124,084	88
Firearm/gunshot	4,084	3	3,331	2	6,569	5	13,984	10
Cut/pierce	615	0	20,775	15	1,500,611	1,058	1,522,001	1,073
Poisoning	6,540	5	128,966	91	543,059	383	678,565	479
Fire/burn	1,589	1	9,450	7	391,349	276	402,389	284
Inhalation/suffocation	3,991	3	4,704	3	32,181	23	40,876	29
Drown/submersion	970	1	1,123	1	974	1	3,067	2
Bite/sting	0	0	13,249	9	1,954,074	1,378	1,967,366	1,387
Natural/environmental	620	0	5,985	4	639,436	451	645,998	456
Overexertion	3	0	19,886	14	2,122,628	1,497	2,142,517	1,511
Other specified	402	0	26,318	19	2,359,353	1,664	2,386,073	1,683
Unspecified	5,065	4	44,340	31	286,878	202	336,283	237

Appendix 1.4 Incidence Counts and Rates (per 100,000) of Motor Vehicle Injuries by Age and Sex, 2000

Age and Sex	Fatal		Hospitalized		Nonhospitalized		Total	
	Incidence	Rate	Incidence	Rate	Incidence	Rate	Incidence	Rate
Total	*43,802*	*16*	*276,183*	*100*	*4,690,454*	*1,697*	*5,010,439*	*1,813*
0–4	835	4	5,307	27	109,168	554	115,310	586
5–14	1,821	4	21,879	53	611,251	1,481	634,950	1,538
15–24	10,534	28	63,020	169	1,186,831	3,177	1,260,385	3,374
25–44	14,053	17	91,480	111	1,769,367	2,141	1,874,899	2,268
45–64	9,001	15	55,677	93	738,140	1,235	802,817	1,343
65–74	3,069	17	17,745	101	170,581	967	191,395	1,085
75+	4,489	30	21,076	140	105,116	694	130,682	863
Male	*29,686*	*22*	*167,893*	*125*	*2,353,751*	*1,749*	*2,551,330*	*1,897*
0–4	463	5	3,038	30	70,399	685	73,900	720
5–14	1,065	5	14,594	70	347,165	1,658	362,824	1,733
15–24	7,474	39	41,030	216	595,296	3,136	643,800	3,392
25–44	10,246	25	59,326	147	887,821	2,202	957,393	2,374
45–64	6,149	21	32,524	113	343,886	1,190	382,559	1,323
65–74	1,824	23	8,334	104	67,216	841	77,373	969
75+	2,465	42	9,048	153	41,968	708	53,482	903
Female	*14,116*	*10*	*108,289*	*76*	*2,336,703*	*1,648*	*2,459,108*	*1,734*
0–4	372	4	2,269	24	38,769	412	41,411	440
5–14	756	4	7,285	36	264,086	1,298	272,126	1,338
15–24	3,060	17	21,990	120	591,535	3,217	616,585	3,353
25–44	3,807	9	32,154	76	881,546	2,083	917,506	2,168
45–64	2,852	9	23,153	75	394,254	1,278	420,259	1,362
65–74	1,245	13	9,411	97	103,365	1,071	114,022	1,181
75+	2,024	22	12,028	130	63,148	685	77,200	837

Appendix 1.5 Incidence Counts and Rates (per 100,000) of Fall Injuries by Age and Sex, 2000

Age and Sex	Fatal		Hospitalized		Nonhospitalized		Total	
	Incidence	Rate	Incidence	Rate	Incidence	Rate	Incidence	Rate
Total	14,052	5	854,589	309	10,698,100	3,870	11,568,382	4,185
0–4	50	0	13,926	71	1,298,889	6,597	1,312,892	6,668
5–14	42	0	25,981	63	2,098,541	5,084	2,124,615	5,147
15–24	359	1	24,084	64	1,126,166	3,014	1,150,657	3,080
25–44	1,194	1	80,331	97	2,255,717	2,729	2,337,399	2,828
45–64	2,011	3	131,793	221	1,905,284	3,188	2,039,342	3,413
65–74	1,701	10	121,850	691	684,953	3,883	808,738	4,585
75+	8,695	57	456,623	3,016	1,328,552	8,775	1,794,740	11,854
Male	7,647	6	306,583	228	4,887,446	3,631	5,202,289	3,865
0–4	33	0	8,094	79	750,578	7,308	758,721	7,388
5–14	32	0	17,181	82	1,179,647	5,633	1,196,895	5,716
15–24	294	2	16,833	89	585,753	3,086	602,914	3,177
25–44	983	2	50,207	125	1,021,204	2,533	1,072,495	2,660
45–64	1,506	5	63,468	220	698,002	2,414	763,103	2,640
65–74	1,018	13	41,388	518	271,882	3,403	314,371	3,935
75+	3,781	64	109,411	1,847	380,382	6,421	493,793	8,335
Female	6,405	5	548,006	386	5,810,654	4,098	6,366,093	4,489
0–4	17	0	5,832	62	548,311	5,823	554,171	5,885
5–14	10	0	8,800	43	918,894	4,518	927,721	4,561
15–24	65	0	7,251	39	540,413	2,939	547,743	2,978
25–44	211	0	30,124	71	1,234,513	2,916	1,264,905	2,988
45–64	505	2	68,325	221	1,207,282	3,913	1,276,240	4,137
65–74	683	7	80,462	834	413,071	4,279	494,367	5,121
75+	4,914	53	347,212	3,766	948,170	10,285	1,300,947	14,111

Appendix 1.6 Incidence Counts and Rate (per 100,000) of Struck by/against Injuries by Age and Sex, 2000

Age and Sex	Fatal		Hospitalized		Nonhospitalized		Total	
	Incidence	Rate	Incidence	Rate	Incidence	Rate	Incidence	Rate
Total	*1,301*	*0*	*85,687*	*31*	*10,759,815*	*3,893*	*10,846,822*	*3,924*
0–4	48	0.2	2,286	12	580,165	2,946	582,499	2,958
5–14	41	0.1	8,675	21	2,714,020	6,575	2,722,738	6,596
15–24	149	0.4	19,271	52	2,669,645	7,146	2,689,068	7,198
25–44	447	0.5	32,413	39	2,940,252	3,557	2,973,118	3,597
45–64	415	0.7	14,682	25	1,411,134	2,361	1,426,234	2,387
65–74	103	0.6	3,167	18	156,241	886	159,511	904
75+	98	0.6	5,195	34	288,358	1,905	293,653	1,940
Male	*1,109*	*0.8*	*66,833*	*50*	*6,675,289*	*4,959*	*6,743,236*	*5,010*
0–4	27	0.3	1,423	14	391,973	3,817	393,423	3,831
5–14	30	0.1	6,825	33	1,939,771	9,263	1,946,627	9,296
15–24	134	0.7	16,453	87	1,673,139	8,815	1,689,727	8,903
25–44	399	1.0	26,833	67	1,750,401	4,341	1,777,635	4,409
45–64	383	1.3	11,529	40	801,198	2,771	813,111	2,813
65–74	80	1.0	1,999	25	84,291	1,055	86,370	1,081
75+	56	0.9	1,770	30	34,516	583	36,342	613
Female	*192*	*0.1*	*18,855*	*13*	*4,084,526*	*2,880*	*4,103,586*	*2,894*
0–4	21	0.2	862	9	188,192	1,999	189,075	2,008
5–14	11	0.1	1,850	9	774,249	3,807	776,111	3,816
15–24	15	0.1	2,818	15	996,506	5,419	999,341	5,434
25–44	48	0.1	5,580	13	1,189,851	2,811	1,195,483	2,824
45–64	32	0.1	3,153	10	609,936	1,977	613,123	1,987
65–74	23	0.2	1,168	12	71,950	745	73,142	758
75+	42	0.5	3,425	37	253,842	2,753	257,311	2,791

Appendix 1.7 Incidence Counts and Rates (per 100,000) of Cut/Pierce Injuries by Age and Sex, 2000

Age and Sex	Fatal		Hospitalized		Nonhospitalized		Total	
	Incidence	Rate	Incidence	Rate	Incidence	Rate	Incidence	Rate
Total	*2,293*	*1*	*71,129*	*26*	*4,104,982*	*1,485*	*4,178,438*	*1,512*
0–4	22	0	1,368	7	140,052	711	141,442	718
5–14	36	0	4,153	10	585,696	1,419	589,887	1,429
15–24	433	1	17,567	47	754,870	2,021	772,878	2,069
25–44	1,078	1	31,829	39	1,704,630	2,062	1,737,552	2,102
45–64	491	1	12,030	20	671,548	1,124	684,075	1,145
65–74	101	1	2,115	12	131,040	743	133,257	755
75+	132	1	2,068	14	117,146	774	119,347	788
Male	*1,678*	*1*	*50,354*	*37*	*2,574,855*	*1,913*	*2,626,906*	*1,952*
0–4	13	0	865	8	94,444	920	95,322	928
5–14	18	0	2,458	12	434,250	2,074	436,727	2,086
15–24	347	2	12,761	67	490,950	2,587	504,062	2,656
25–44	779	2	22,886	57	1,113,706	2,762	1,137,380	2,821
45–64	359	1	8,783	30	295,178	1,021	304,323	1,053
65–74	72	1	1,465	18	102,054	1,277	103,591	1,297
75+	90	2	1,137	19	44,273	747	45,501	768
Female	*615*	*0*	*20,775*	*15*	*1,530,127*	*1,079*	*1,551,531*	*1,094*
0–4	9	0	503	5	45,608	484	46,120	490
5–14	18	0	1,695	8	151,446	745	153,160	753
15–24	86	0	4,806	26	263,920	1,435	268,815	1,462
25–44	299	1	8,943	21	590,924	1,396	600,172	1,418
45–64	132	0	3,247	11	376,370	1,220	379,752	1,231
65–74	29	0	650	7	28,986	300	29,665	307
75+	42	0	931	10	72,873	790	73,846	801

Appendix 1.8 Incidence Counts and Rates (per 100,000) of Fire/Burn Injuries by Age and Sex, 2000

Age and Sex	Fatal		Hospitalized		Nonhospitalized		Total	
	Incidence	Rate	Incidence	Rate	Incidence	Rate	Incidence	Rate
Total	*3,922*	*1*	*24,519*	*9*	*745,935*	*270*	*774,376*	*280*
0–4	371	2	3,416	17	104,247	529	108,034	549
5–14	297	1	1,627	4	50,399	122	52,323	127
15–24	241	1	2,538	7	121,363	325	124,142	332
25–44	821	1	7,087	9	174,745	211	182,653	221
45–64	930	2	5,507	9	226,690	379	233,127	390
65–74	443	3	1,911	11	35,743	203	38,097	216
75+	819	5	2,432	16	32,748	216	35,999	238
Male	*2,333*	*2*	*15,069*	*11*	*354,586*	*263*	*371,988*	*276*
0–4	220	2	1,908	19	65,716	640	67,844	661
5–14	163	1	1,037	5	25,354	121	26,554	127
15–24	146	1	1,880	10	80,116	422	82,142	433
25–44	531	1	4,732	12	101,910	253	107,173	266
45–64	615	2	3,404	12	71,258	246	75,277	260
65–74	262	3	1,080	14	6,264	78	7,606	95
75+	396	7	1,027	17	3,967	67	5,390	91
Female	*1,589*	*1*	*9,450*	*7*	*391,349*	*276*	*402,389*	*284*
0–4	151	2	1,508	16	38,531	409	40,190	427
5–14	134	1	590	3	25,045	123	25,769	127
15–24	95	1	658	4	41,247	224	42,000	228
25–44	290	1	2,355	6	72,835	172	75,480	178
45–64	315	1	2,103	7	155,432	504	157,850	512
65–74	181	2	831	9	29,479	305	30,491	316
75+	423	5	1,405	15	28,780	312	30,609	332

Appendix 1.9 Incidence Counts and Rates (per 100,000) of Drowning/Submersion Injuries by Age and Sex, 2000

	Fatal		Hospitalized		Nonhospitalized		Total	
Age and Sex	Incidence	Rate	Incidence	Rate	Incidence	Rate	Incidence	Rate
Total	*4,168*	*2*	*3,289*	*1*	*2,627*	*1*	*10,100*	*4*
0–4	601	3	1,022	5	1,619	8	3,248	16
5–14	386	1	580	1	489	1	1,457	4
15–24	746	2	395	1	189	1	1,332	4
25–44	1,129	1	661	1	231	0	2,023	2
45–64	743	1	376	1	0	0	1,122	2
65–74	239	1	150	1	0	0	390	2
75+	324	2	105	1	99	1	528	3
Male	*3,198*	*2*	*2,166*	*2*	*1,652*	*1*	*7,026*	*5*
0–4	372	4	633	6	1,074	10	2,083	20
5–14	272	1	334	2	288	1	895	4
15–24	664	3	290	2	59	0	1,015	5
25–44	941	2	480	1	231	1	1,654	4
45–64	591	2	259	1	0	0	852	3
65–74	169	2	103	1	0	0	272	3
75+	189	3	67	1	0	0	256	4
Female	*970*	*1*	*1,123*	*1*	*974*	*1*	*3,073*	*2*
0–4	229	2	389	4	545	6	1,166	12
5–14	114	1	246	1	201	1	562	3
15–24	82	0	105	1	130	1	317	2
25–44	188	0	181	0	0	0	370	1
45–64	152	0	117	0	0	0	270	1
65–74	70	1	47	0	0	0	118	1
75+	135	1	38	0	99	1	272	3

Appendix 1.10 Incidence Counts and Rates (per 100,000) of Poisoning Injuries by Age and Sex, 2000

Age and Sex	Fatal		Hospitalized		Nonhospitalized		Total	
	Incidence	Rate	Incidence	Rate	Incidence	Rate	Incidence	Rate
Total	*20,261*	*7*	*219,056*	*79*	*1,028,148*	*372*	*1,267,465*	*459*
0–4	63	0	6,487	33	148,823	756	155,372	789
5–14	78	0	7,523	18	56,651	137	64,252	156
15–24	1,671	4	44,791	120	276,100	739	322,562	863
25–44	10,814	13	94,302	114	258,294	313	363,410	440
45–64	6,352	11	44,734	75	109,511	183	160,598	269
65–74	540	3	9,374	53	163,058	924	172,972	981
75+	743	5	11,845	78	15,709	104	28,297	187
Male	*13,721*	*10*	*90,090*	*67*	*485,089*	*360*	*588,900*	*438*
0–4	42	0	3,596	35	108,152	1,053	111,790	1,089
5–14	49	0	2,185	10	12,076	58	14,310	68
15–24	1,269	7	16,515	87	64,062	338	81,846	431
25–44	7,599	19	40,333	100	164,805	409	212,737	528
45–64	4,122	14	19,603	68	77,643	269	101,368	351
65–74	275	3	3,671	46	48,920	612	52,866	662
75+	365	6	4,187	71	9,429	159	13,982	236
Female	*6,540*	*5*	*128,966*	*91*	*543,059*	*383*	*678,565*	*479*
0–4	21	0	2,891	31	40,671	432	43,583	463
5–14	29	0	5,338	26	44,575	219	49,942	246
15–24	402	2	28,276	154	212,038	1,153	240,716	1,309
25–44	3,215	8	53,969	127	93,489	221	150,673	356
45–64	2,230	7	25,131	81	31,868	103	59,229	192
65–74	265	3	5,703	59	114,138	1,182	120,106	1,244
75+	378	4	7,658	83	6,280	68	14,316	155

Appendix 1.11 Incidence Counts and Rates (per 100,000) of Firearm/Gunshot Injuries by Age and Sex, 2000

Age and Sex	Fatal		Hospitalized		Nonhospitalized		Total	
	Incidence	Rate	Incidence	Rate	Incidence	Rate	Incidence	Rate
Total	28,722	10	29,609	11	72,682	26	131,298	48
0–4	59	0	220	1	405	2	687	3
5–14	377	1	1,279	3	30,198	73	31,869	77
15–24	6,593	18	12,946	35	22,241	60	41,889	112
25–44	11,182	14	11,982	14	16,484	20	39,762	48
45–64	6,228	10	2,554	4	3,069	5	11,885	20
65–74	1,942	11	353	2	284	2	2,585	15
75+	2,341	15	275	2	0	0	2,621	17
Male	24,638	18	26,278	20	66,113	49	117,171	87
0–4	37	0	163	2	290	3	491	5
5–14	302	1	1,085	5	28,501	136	29,894	143
15–24	5,924	31	11,928	63	19,620	103	37,537	198
25–44	9,399	23	10,647	26	14,905	37	35,009	87
45–64	5,158	18	2,021	7	2,538	9	9,728	34
65–74	1,685	21	251	3	259	3	2,196	27
75+	2,133	36	183	3	0	0	2,317	39
Female	4,084	3	3,331	2	6,569	5	14,126	10
0–4	22	0	57	1	115	1	197	2
5–14	75	0	194	1	1,697	8	1,975	10
15–24	669	4	1,018	6	2,621	14	4,352	24
25–44	1,783	4	1,335	3	1,579	4	4,753	11
45–64	1,070	3	533	2	531	2	2,157	7
65–74	257	3	102	1	25	0	388	4
75+	208	2	92	1	0	0	304	3

Chapter 2

Lifetime Medical Costs of Injuries

Every year, injuries impose a significant financial burden on the U.S. health care system. For some injuries, medical treatment and corresponding costs may persist for years or even decades after the initial injury. This chapter combines incidence counts from the previous chapter with the unit cost of medical treatment and rehabilitation to estimate the lifetime costs for medically treated injuries that occurred in 2000. Due to data limitations, the medical costs presented in this chapter include costs associated with treatment for physical injuries only; data required to estimate costs for mental health and psychological treatment were not available.

As with Chapter 1, the cost estimates presented in this chapter are divided into three mutually exclusive categories that reflect the severity of injury: (1) injury resulting in death, including deaths occurring within and outside a healthcare setting; (2) injury resulting in hospitalization with survival to discharge; and (3) injury requiring medical attention without hospitalization. The latter category includes injuries requiring an emergency department visit, an office-based visit, or a hospital outpatient visit. Injuries that were not severe enough to require medical attention are not included in our calculations. We sum the cost of injuries across these mutually exclusive categories to quantify total lifetime medical costs. Additional tables, including several that provide unit cost estimates not included in the body of the chapter, are presented in an appendix.

For each injury category (i.e., fatal, hospitalized, nonhospitalized), total medical costs are stratified by the following:

- Age and sex (for males and females in the following age categories: 0–4, 5–14, 15–24, 25–44, 45–64, 65–74, or 75 and older);

- Mechanism of injury (including motor vehicle/other road user, falls, struck by/against, cut/pierce, fire/burn, poisoning, drowning/submersion, firearm/gunshot, or other);
- Body region (including traumatic brain injury, other head/neck, spinal cord injury, vertebral column injury, torso, upper extremity, lower extremity, other/unspecified, or system-wide based on the Barell Injury Diagnosis Matrix);
- Severity of injury (based on the Abbreviated Injury Score [AIS]); and
- Nature of injury (including fracture, dislocation, sprain/strain, internal organ, open wound, amputation, blood vessel, superficial/contusion, crushing, burn, nerve, system-wide, or unspecified).

In addition, total and unit medical costs for injuries that result from eight major mechanisms are examined by age and sex. All cost estimates are reported in 2000 dollars. Specifics regarding the data and methods used to develop these cost estimates are described at the end of the chapter.

Total Lifetime Medical Costs of Injuries

Table 2.1 presents total lifetime medical costs for injuries that occurred in 2000 by age and sex. Corresponding unit cost estimates are presented in Appendix Table 2.1. Ultimately, injuries that occurred in 2000 will cost the U.S. health care system $80.2 billion in medical care costs: $1.1 billion for fatal injuries; $33.7 billion for hospitalized injuries; and $45.4 billion for nonhospitalized injuries, with 70% ($31.8 billion) of the nonhospitalized costs attributable to injuries treated in the emergency department (see Appendix Table 2.3). Figure 2.1 compares the distribution of injury incidence to the distribution of total medical costs across three mutually exclusive categories (i.e., fatal, hospitalized, nonhospitalized). Injury hospitalizations, which accounted for nearly 4% of all injuries in 2000, represent 42% of injury-attributable medical costs. Not only are hospitalized injuries more expensive to treat in the short-term, but they may require long-term rehabilitation, further contributing to lifetime costs. In contrast, nonhospitalized injuries, which accounted for 96% of all injuries, represent only 57% of injury-attributable medical costs.

Injuries among males account for $44.4 billion, or approximately 55% of all medical costs for injuries; injuries among females account for $35.8 billion, or approximately 45% of all medical costs for injuries. This cost distribution is similar to the incidence distribution reported in Chapter 1: males accounted for 53% of injuries, while females accounted for 47% of injuries.

Figure 2.2 compares the distribution of injury incidence to the distribution of total injury-attributable medical costs by age group. Those aged 25 to 44 years account for $22.7 billion, or approximately 30% of injury-attributable medical costs. This age group also represents 30% of the U.S. population and accounted for 30% of all injuries. In contrast, those aged greater than 75 years (representing 5% of the population) accounted for only 6% of all injuries, yet they represent 16% (or $12.6 billion) of the medical costs for injuries. In Figure 2.3, 79% of injury-attributable medical costs among people aged 75 years and older result from fatal (3%) and hospitalized injuries (76%). In contrast, only 15% of the medical costs for injuries among people aged 5 to 14 years result from fatal (<1%) and hospitalized injuries (14.6 %).

Table 2.1 Total Lifetime Medical Costs of Injuries by Age and Sex, 2000 ($M)

	Fatal	Hospitalized	Nonhospitalized	Total
All	*$1,113*	*$33,738*	*$45,398*	*$80,248*
0–4	28	595	3,107	3,729
5–14	35	1,191	6,944	8,170
15–24	108	4,405	8,382	12,895
25–44	223	7,881	14,599	22,704
45–64	215	6,483	7,580	14,278
65–74	116	3,615	2,134	5,865
75+	386	9,569	2,653	12,608
Male	*$683*	*$18,531*	*$25,231*	*$44,445*
0–4	16	359	2,063	2,438
5–14	22	784	4,166	4,973
15–24	83	3,271	4,992	8,346
25–44	168	5,625	8,240	14,033
45–64	151	4,024	3,824	7,999
65–74	69	1,597	1,038	2,704
75+	174	2,871	907	3,952
Female	*$429*	*$15,207*	*$20,168*	*$35,804*
0–4	11	236	1,044	1,291
5–14	13	406	2,778	3,197
15–24	25	1,133	3,391	4,549
25–44	56	2,256	6,359	8,671
45–64	65	2,459	3,755	6,279
65–74	47	2,018	1,096	3,160
75+	212	6,698	1,746	8,656

Incidence

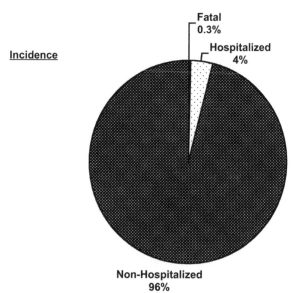

**Fatal
0.3%**

**Hospitalized
4%**

**Non-Hospitalized
96%**

Figure 2.1a Distribution of
Injury Incidence by Injury
Category, 2000

58

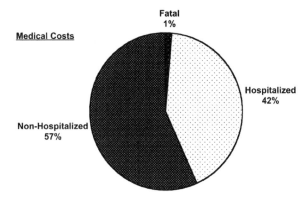

Fatal
1%

Hospitalized
42%

Non-Hospitalized
57%

Figure 2.1b Distribution
of Total Lifetime Medical
Costs of Injuries by Injury
Category, 2000

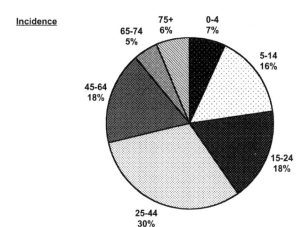

Incidence

75+
6%

65-74
5%

0-4
7%

5-14
16%

45-64
18%

15-24
18%

25-44
30%

Figure 2.2a Distribution
of Injury Incidence by Age
Group, 2000

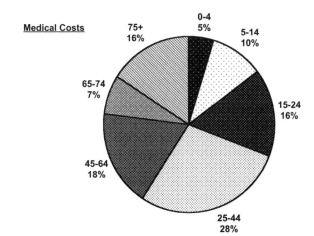

Medical Costs

0-4
5%

75+
16%

5-14
10%

65-74
7%

15-24
16%

45-64
18%

25-44
28%

Figure 2.2b Distribution of
Total Lifetime Medical Costs of
Injuries by Age Group, 2000

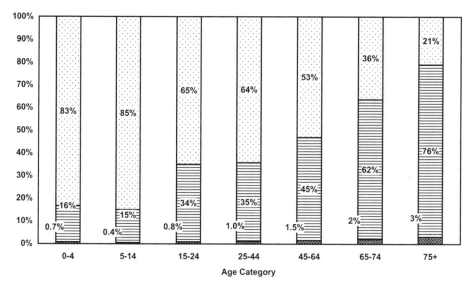

■ Fatal ▣ Hospitalized ☐ Non Hospitalized

Figure 2.3 Distribution of Total Lifetime Medical Costs of Injuries by Age Group and In-jury Category, 2000

Conversely, the percentage of medical costs attributable to nonhospitalized injuries decreases as age increases (Figure 2.3).

Age and Sex Patterns

Figure 2.4 shows total lifetime medical costs by age group and sex. For age groups younger than 65, males account for a greater percentage of injury-attributable medical costs than females. In fact, injury-attributable medical costs for males aged 0 to 4 ($2.4 billion) and 15 to 24 years ($8.3 billion) are 89% and 83% higher than injury-attributable medical costs for same-age females. However, for age groups older than 65, females account for a greater percentage of injury-attributable medical costs than males. Medical costs for injuries among females aged 75 years and older ($8.7 billion) are more than double the total medical costs for injuries among same-age males ($4.0 billion).

Figure 2.5 shows total lifetime medical costs for fatal, hospitalized, and nonhos-pitalized injuries by age group and sex. For fatal injuries, medical costs for males are higher than those for females for all age groups younger than 75. This pattern is largely driven by the incidence of fatal injuries; for all age groups younger than 75, males account for a greater number of fatal injuries than females (Chapter 1). The male to female ratio of medical costs for fatal injuries is nearly identical to the male to female ratio of incidence for fatal injuries for all age categories up to age 64 years, with males accounting for a higher percentage of both medical costs and incidence. In contrast, females aged 65 to 74 and 75 and older (relative to same-aged males) ac-count for 41% and 55% of injury-attributable medical costs for fatal injuries, but

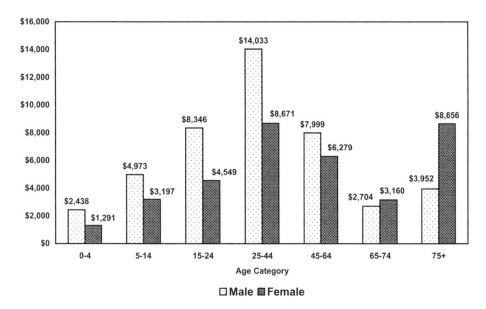

Figure 2.4 Total Lifetime Medical Costs of Injuries by Age Group and Sex, 2000 ($M)

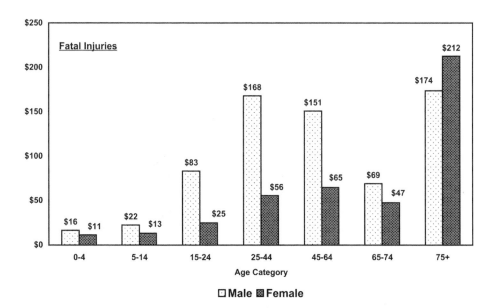

Figure 2.5a Total Lifetime Medical Costs of Fatal Injuries by Age Group and Sex, 2000 ($M)

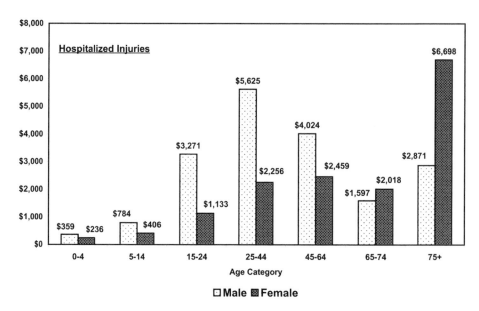

Figure 2.5b Total Lifetime Medical Costs of Hospitalized Injuries by Age Group and Sex, 2000 ($M)

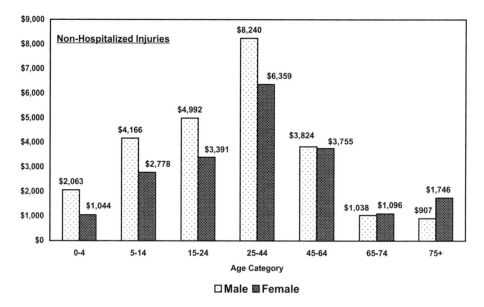

Figure 2.5c Total Lifetime Medical Costs of Nonhospitalized Injuries by Age Group and Sex, 2000 ($M)

only 35% and 50% of the incidence for fatal injuries (Chapter 1). Appendix Table 2.1 provides the corresponding unit cost estimates.

For hospitalized injuries, males account for a greater percentage of attributable medical costs than do females for all age groups younger than 65. Comparing the distribution of injury-attributable medical costs with that of injury incidence, except for males aged 0 to 4 and 5 to 14 years, males account for a greater percentage of medical costs for hospitalized injuries than they account for the incidence of hospitalized injuries (relative to same-aged females). In particular, males aged 15 to 24, 25 to 44, and 45 to 64 years account for 74%, 71%, and 62% of the medical costs for hospitalized injuries, but only 65%, 63%, and 54% of the incidence of hospitalized injuries (Chapter 1). This may indicate that hospitalized injuries among males in these age groups are, on average, more severe or more difficult to treat than injuries among same-aged females. For nonhospitalized injuries, the medical cost distribution between males and females in all age groups is nearly identical to the corresponding incidence distribution (Chapter 1).

Total Lifetime Medical Costs by Mechanism

Table 2.2 presents total lifetime medical costs of injuries by mechanism and sex. Treatment for falls ($26.9 billion) and motor-vehicle crashes ($14 billion) represent roughly half of injury-attributable medical costs ($80.2 billion). Yet, these two mechanisms represent only one third of injury incidence. Figure 2.6 compares the distribution of injury incidence to the distribution of total lifetime medical costs by mechanism. Several mechanisms, including falls and motor vehicles, represent a disproportionate fraction of total medical costs. Falls and motor vehicle injuries, which accounted for 23% and 10% of all injuries in 2000, represent 34% and 17% of medical costs of injuries. The high cost of motor vehicle injuries results from their severity relative to other types of injuries. Falls are more likely to occur among the elderly, which increases treatment costs. In contrast, struck by/against injuries, which accounted for 22% of all injuries in 2000, represent only 14% of medical costs of injuries.

Figure 2.7 shows the distribution of injury-attributable total lifetime medical costs by injury category (i.e., fatal, hospitalized, nonhospitalized) and mechanism. Motor vehicle/other road users and falls account for approximately half of the medical costs of fatal injuries, 31% and 21%, respectively. These same two mechanisms account for more than two thirds of the medical costs of hospitalized injuries; falls alone represent 45% of this total, and motor vehicles represent an additional 24%. For nonhospitalized injuries, falls, struck by/against, and motor-vehicle injuries account for 25%, 21%, and 12% of injury-attributable medical costs.

Figure 2.8 compares total lifetime medical costs of injuries by sex and mechanism. With the exception of falls (44%) and poisonings (48%), males account for more than half of the medical costs associated with each injury mechanism. The medical costs associated with struck by/against and cut/pierce injuries among males are double those for females; the medical costs associated with firearm/gunshot injuries among males are more than 7 times those for females. These cost disparities, however, are largely driven by a higher incidence of these injuries among males. The

Table 2.2 Total Lifetime Medical Costs of Injuries by Mechanism and Sex, 2000 ($M)

	Fatal	Hospitalized	Nonhospitalized	Total
All	*$1,113*	*$33,737*	*$45,398*	*$80,248*
MV/other road user	$342	$8,200	$5,484	$14,026
Falls	232	15,247	11,413	26,892
Struck by/against	12	1,474	9,542	11,028
Cut/pierce	11	732	2,919	3,662
Fire/burn	66	461	817	1,345
Poisoning	73	1,408	756	2,236
Drowning/submersion	13	78	4	95
Firearm/gunshot	85	1,089	52	1,225
Other	279	5,047	14,412	19,738
Male	*$683*	*$18,531*	*$25,231*	*$44,445*
MV/other road user	$225	$5,473	$3,015	$8,713
Falls	122	6,260	5,396	11,778
Struck by/against	10	1,204	6,279	7,493
Cut/pierce	9	565	1,868	2,442
Fire/burn	37	297	430	764
Poison	43	625	396	1,063
Drowning/submersion	9	49	3	61
Firearm/gunshot	74	961	46	1,081
Other	155	3,097	7,798	11,050
Female	*$429*	*$15,206*	*$20,168*	*$35,803*
MV/other road user	$118	$2,727	$2,468	$5,313
Falls	110	8,988	6,016	15,114
Struck by/against	2	269	3,264	3,535
Cut/pierce	2	167	1,051	1,221
Fire/burn	28	165	387	581
Poison	30	783	360	1,173
Drowning/submersion	4	29	1	34
Firearm/gunshot	11	127	6	144
Other	125	1,950	6,614	8,688

incidence of struck by/against and cut/pierce injuries among males is nearly double that among females; the incidence of firearm/gunshot injuries among males is more than 8 times that among females (Chapter 1).

Figure 2.9 compares total lifetime medical costs of fatal, hospitalized, and non-hospitalized injuries by sex and mechanism. For fatal injuries, males account for more than 50% of the medical costs of each injury mechanism, and more than 75% of the medical costs of firearm/gunshot, struck by/against, and cut/pierce injuries. For hospitalized injuries, females account for more than 50% of injury-attributable medical costs of falls (59%) and poisonings (56%), while males account for more than 60% of injury-attributable medical costs for all other mechanisms. The distribution of medical costs of hospitalized firearm/gunshot, struck by/against, and

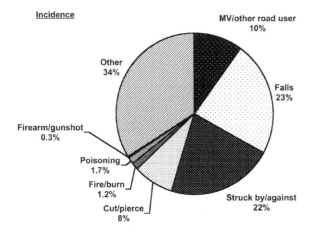

Figure 2.6a Distribution of Injury Incidence by Mechanism, 2000

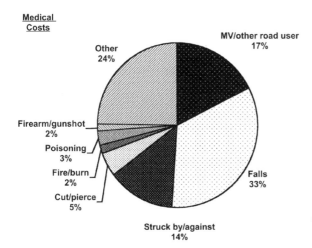

Figure 2.6b Distribution of Total Lifetime Medical Costs of Injuries by Mechanism, 2000

cut/pierce injuries is almost identical to that of fatal injuries, with men accounting for 88%, 82%, and 77%, respectively. For less severe injuries (i.e., nonhospitalized injuries), medical costs by mechanism are more evenly distributed between males and females, with the exception of firearm/gunshot injuries, for which males account for 88% of total medical costs, and struck by/against injuries, for which males account for 66% of total medical costs.

Total Lifetime Medical Costs by Body Region, Severity, and Nature of Injury

Table 2.3 presents total lifetime medical costs of injuries by body region. Corresponding unit cost estimates are presented in Appendix Table 2.5. Combined, upper-extremity ($16.9 billion) and lower-extremity ($24.2 billion) injuries account

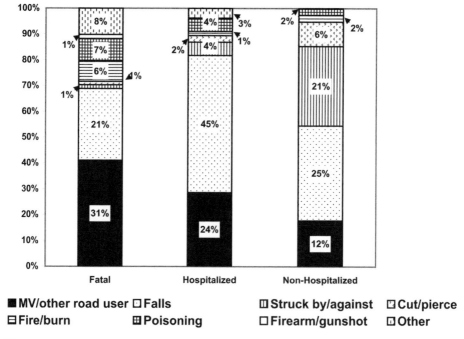

Figure 2.7 Distribution of Total Lifetime Medical Costs by Injury Category and Mechanism

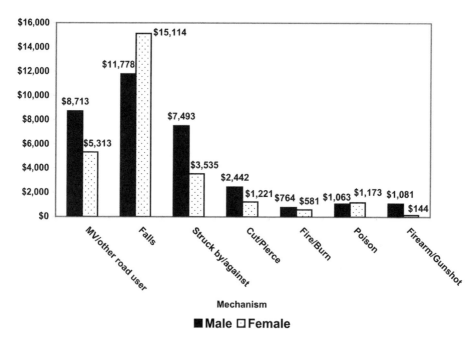

Figure 2.8 Total Lifetime Medical Costs of Injuries by Sex and Mechanism, 2000 ($M)

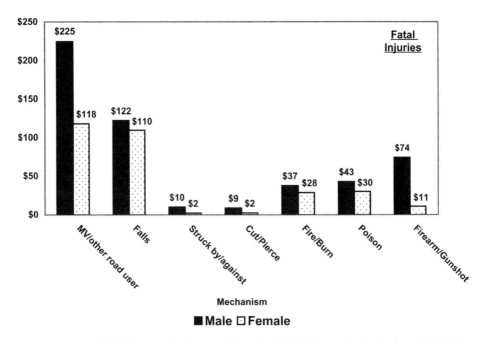

Figure 2.9a Total Lifetime Medical Costs of Fatal Injuries by Sex and Mechanism, 2000 ($M)

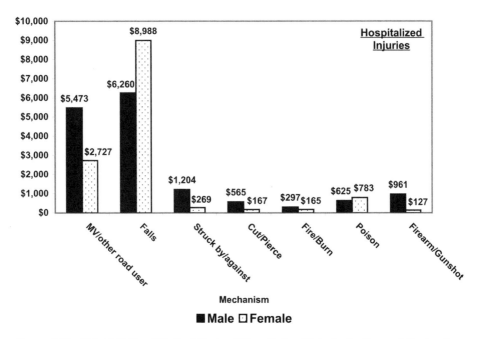

Figure 2.9b Total Lifetime Medical Costs of Hospitalized Injuries by Sex and Mechanism, 2000 ($M)

67

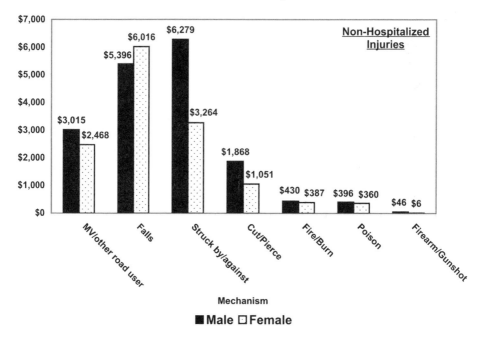

Figure 2.9c Total Lifetime Medical Costs of Nonhospitalized Injuries by Sex and Mechanism, 2000 ($M)

for more than 50% of medical costs of injuries. Figure 2.10 compares the distribution of injuries to the distribution of injury-attributable medical costs by body region. Relative to incidence, a disproportionate fraction of medical costs are allocated to traumatic brain and spinal cord injuries. These injuries, which accounted for 3% and 0.1% of all injuries in 2000, account for 11% ($9.2 billion) and 2% ($1.6 billion) of injury-attributable medical costs. Much of this total, 80% and 97%, is associated with hospitalized injuries, which indicates the increased severity of trau-

Table 2.3 Total Lifetime Medical Costs of Injuries by Body Region, 2000 ($M)

Body Region	Fatal	Hospitalized	Nonhospitalized	Total
All	$1,113	$33,737	$45,398	$80,248
Traumatic brain injury	336	7,377	1,509	9,222
Other head/neck	36	1,663	4,683	6,382
Spinal cord injury	13	1,588	29	1,629
Vertebral column injury	10	1,073	4,626	5,709
Torso	189	3,532	3,126	6,847
Upper extremity	9	3,183	13,749	16,941
Lower extremity	132	12,491	11,612	24,236
Other/unspecified	245	223	4,270	4,738
System-wide	144	2,605	1,794	4,544

Incidence

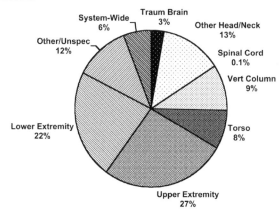

Figure 2.10a Distribution of Injury Incidence by Body Region, 2000

matic brain and spinal cord injuries. The relatively high medical costs of these injuries result, in part, from the need for long term care and rehabilitation.

Table 2.4 presents total lifetime medical costs of injuries by nature of injury. Corresponding unit cost estimates are presented in Appendix Table 2.6. Fractures ($27.4 billion) and strains/sprains ($15.3 billion) account for more than 50% of the medical costs of injuries. Table 2.5 compares the distribution of injuries to the distribution of injury-attributable medical costs by nature of injury. Fracture and internal organ injuries, which represented 14% and <2% of all injuries in 2000, represent 34% and 9% of the medical costs of injuries. In contrast, sprain/strain, superficial/contusion, and open-wound injuries, which represented 30%, 21%, and 18% of all injuries in 2000, are only 19%, 11%, and 10% of injury-attributable medical costs.

Figure 2.11 indicates that medical costs associated with the less severe AIS 1 and 2 injuries ($32 billon and $19 billion, respectively) constitute 85% of cases (see Chapter 1) but represent only 63.4% of the total medical costs. This difference can be explained by the lower medical cost per episode for less severe injuries. Conversely, the

Medical Costs

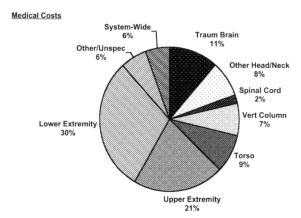

Figure 2.10b Distribution of Total Lifetime Medical Costs of Injuries by Body Region, 2000

Table 2.4 Total Lifetime Medical Costs of Injuries by Nature of Injury, 2000 ($M)

Nature of Injury	Fatal	Hospitalized	Nonhospitalized	Total
All	*1,113*	*33,737*	*34,849*	*80,248*
Fracture	184	19,032	19,216	27,407
Dislocation	2	318	320	2,856
Sprain/strain	0	980	980	15,260
Internal organ	170	6,864	7,034	7,528
Open wound	90	1,472	1,562	8,033
Amputation	0	130	130	189
Blood Vessel	55	173	228	245
Superficial/contusion	4	1,303	1,307	8,559
Crushing	3	40	43	320
Burn	7	418	425	1,337
Nerve	1	111	112	194
Unspecified	452	292	744	3,776
System-wide	144	2,605	2,750	4,544

most severe nonfatal injuries (AIS 4 and 5) have high medical expenses. These 0.4% of cases account for 9.7% ($7.9 billion) of total medical costs.

Medical Cost Patterns by Mechanism

The following section describes unit and total lifetime medical costs of injuries, separately for eight major mechanisms. Medical costs are stratified by age group and sex. Unit and total injury-attributable medical costs of more detailed mechanism categories are provided in Appendix Table 2.2 and Appendix Table 2.3. Figure 2.12 shows the distribution of total lifetime medical costs of fatal, hospitalized, and non-hospitalized injuries by mechanism.

Table 2.5 Distribution of Injuries and Total Lifetime Medical Costs of Injuries by Nature of Injury, 2000

Nature of Injury	Distribution of Injuries (%)	Distribution of Costs (%)
Fracture	14	34
Dislocation	3	4
Sprain/strain	30	19
Internal organ	1	9
Open wound	18	10
Amputation	0.1	0.2
Blood vessel	0.0	0.3
Superficial/contusion	21	11
Crushing	0.4	0.4
Burn	2	2
Nerve	0.2	0.2
Unspecified	5	5
System-wide	6	6

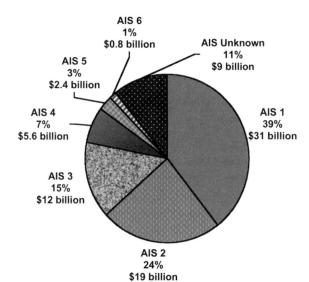

Figure 2.11 Distribution of Total Lifetime Medical Costs by Severity, 2000

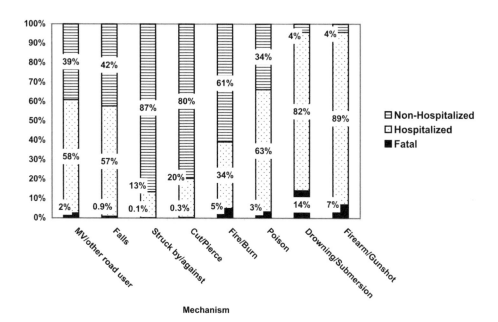

Figure 2.12 Distribution of Total Lifetime Medical Costs of Fatal, Hospitalized, and Non-hospitalized Injuries by Mechanism, 2000

Motor Vehicle/Other Road User

Roughly 17%, or $14 billion, of injury-attributable medical costs result from motor-vehicle crashes (Table 2.2). Fatal and hospitalized injuries, as indicated in Figure 2.12, account for 60% of this total.

Figure 2.13 shows unit and total lifetime medical costs of motor-vehicle injuries by age and sex. Regardless of age, unit medical costs are greater for males than females. These higher unit-cost estimates are driven by the increased incidence of fatal and hospitalized motor-vehicle injuries that occur among males (Chapter 1). For both males and females, persons 75 years and older account for the highest unit medical costs, $6,009 and $4,417, respectively. However, because the elderly are involved in a relatively small number of motor-vehicle injuries, they account for less than 5% of total motor-vehicle/other road-user-attributable medical costs. Males and females aged 25 to 44 years, on the other hand, accrue more than a third of the total injury-attributable medical costs for motor-vehicle injuries, $3.2 billion and $1.8 billion, respectively.

Falls

At 34%, or $26.9 billion, falls represent a greater percentage of injury-attributable medical costs than any other injury mechanism. Similar to the cost distribution for motor-vehicle accidents, fatal and hospitalized injuries, as indicated in Figure 2.12, account for nearly 58% of total fall-related medical costs.

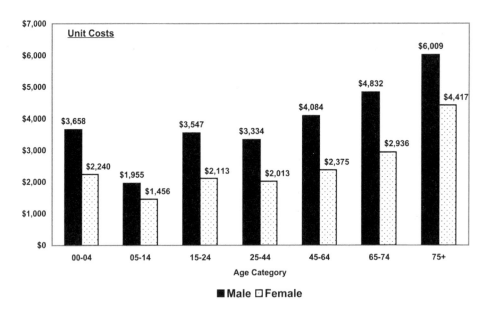

Figure 2.13a Unit Medical Costs of Motor-Vehicle–Related Injuries by Sex and Age Group, 2000

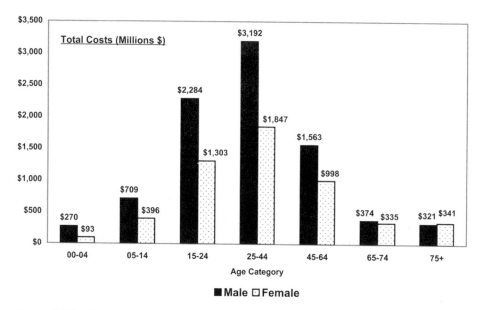

Figure 2.13b Total Medical Costs ($M) of Motor-Vehicle–Related Injuries by Sex and Age Group, 2000

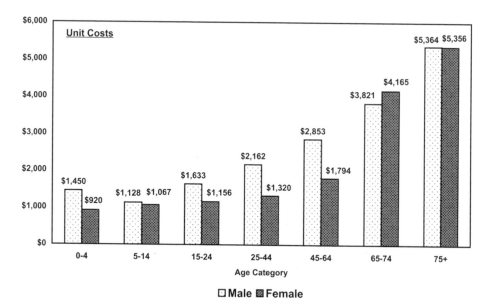

Figure 2.14a Unit Costs of Fall-Related Injuries by Sex and Age Group, 2000

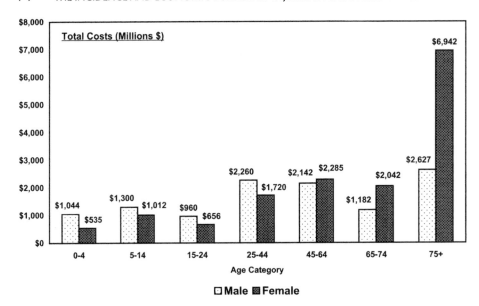

Figure 2.14b Total Medical Costs ($M) of Fall-Related Injuries by Sex and Age Group, 2000

Figure 2.14 shows unit and total lifetime medical costs of fall-related injuries by age and sex. In general, unit medical costs of falls increase as age increases. Although the circumstances leading to the fall may be different for each age group, the adverse health effects of any type of fall likely increase with age. As a result, males and females aged 75 years and older account for higher average unit medical costs than any other age group, $5,364 and $5,356, respectively. Although those aged 75 years and older represent only 5% of the total U.S. population, they accounted for 62% and 53% of the fatal and hospitalized fall incidence (Chapter 1). In fact, by themselves, females aged 75 years and older represent approximately 26% of the total medical costs of fall-related injuries.

Struck by/against

Approximately 14%, or $11 billion, of injury-attributable medical costs result from struck by/against injuries (Table 2.2). Unlike the cost distributions for motor-vehicle accidents and falls, fatal and hospitalized injuries account for less than 14% of the medical costs of struck by/against injuries (Figure 2.12).

Figure 2.15 shows unit and total lifetime medical costs of struck by/against injuries by age and sex. For all age groups, other than persons aged 0 to 4 years, males have higher unit medical costs than females. These higher unit cost estimates are likely driven, in part, by the increased incidence of hospitalized struck by/against injuries among males for all age groups up to age 75 (Chapter 1). The disparity between males and females is greatest among those aged 75 years and older, with unit costs of $1,764 and $950, respectively. However, because the incidence of struck by/against injuries among females in this age group is almost 5 times that among

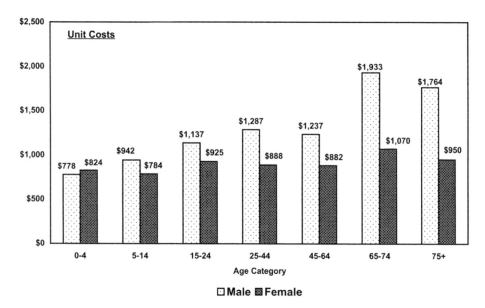

Figure 2.15a Unit Costs of Struck by/against Injuries by Sex and Age Group, 2000

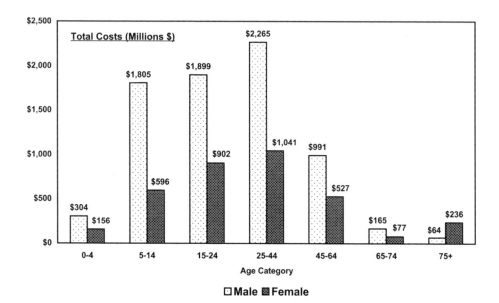

Figure 2.15b Total Medical Costs ($M) of Struck by/against Injuries by Sex and Age Group, 2000

same-aged males, total injury-attributable medical costs for females 75 years and older are actually higher ($236 million) than those for males of the same age ($64 million). Conversely, because the incidence of struck by/against injuries is higher among males for all other age categories, total injury-attributable medical costs are higher among males for all other age categories as well.

Cut/Pierce

Roughly 5%, or $3.7 billion, of injury-attributable medical costs result from cut/pierce injuries (Table 2.2). As shown in Figure 2.12, nonhospitalized injuries account for the majority (80%) of the medical costs of cut/pierce injuries.

Figure 2.16 shows unit and total lifetime medical costs of cut/pierce injuries by age group and sex. For males, unit medical costs range from $678 for those aged 5 to 14 years to $1,208 for those aged 45 to 64 years. This cost disparity is largely explained by typical treatment location (e.g., injuries seen in a hospital versus an emergency department [ED] versus a doctor's office). Among males aged 5 to 14 years, approximately 50% of cut/pierce injuries are treated in hospitals or EDs, while among males aged 45 to 64 years, more than 90% of cut/pierce injuries are treated in hospitals or EDs. An increased likelihood of treatment in hospitals or EDs is indicative of increased injury severity. For females, unit medical costs range from $682 for those aged 75 years and older, to $1,114 for those aged 65 to 74 years. Similar to the findings for males, higher unit medical costs are driven by a higher incidence of cut/pierce injuries treated in hospitals and EDs.

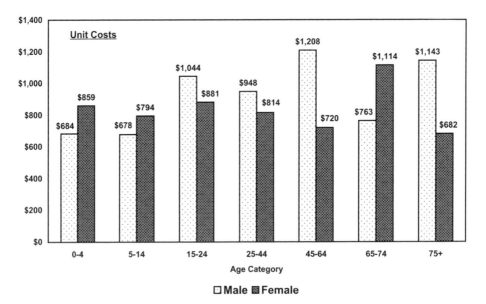

Figure 2.16a Unit Costs of Cut/Pierce Injuries by Sex and Age Group, 2000

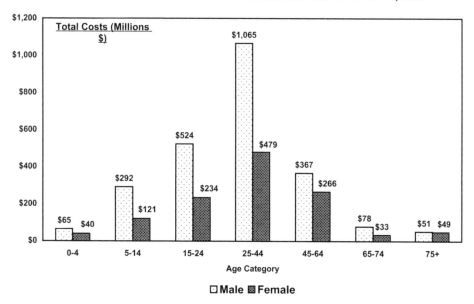

Figure 2.16b Total Medical Costs ($M) of Cut/Pierce Injuries by Sex and Age Group, 2000

Fire/Burns

Fire/burn injuries account for less than 2% ($1.3 billion) of medical costs for all injuries; however, they account for 6% ($66 million) of medical costs for fatal injuries (Table 2.2).

Figure 2.17 shows unit and total lifetime medical costs of fire/burn injuries by age and sex. Unit medical costs for males and females are similar for all age groups younger than 45. For those 45 years and older, unit medical costs for males are higher than those for females. The primary reason for this disparity is the relatively high incidence of nonhospitalized fire/burn injuries among females (Chapter 1). Because these less severe injuries typically have lower treatment costs than fatal or hospitalized fire/burn injuries, the unit medical costs for females are less than that for males. For both males ($256 million) and females ($168 million), those aged 25 to 44 years have the highest total injury-attributable medical costs of fire/burn injuries.

Poisoning

Poisonings, at roughly $2.2 billion, account for less than 3% of injury-attributable medical costs, and 7% ($73 million) and 4% ($1.4 billion) of the medical costs of fatal and hospitalized injuries (Table 2.2). Although less than 20% of poisonings result in fatalities or hospitalizations, these relatively severe injuries account for more than 65% of the total medical costs of poisonings (Figure 2.12).

Figure 2.18 shows unit and total lifetime medical costs of poisoning injuries by age and sex. In general, unit medical costs of poisonings increase as age increases,

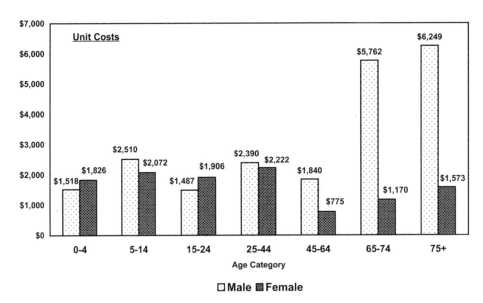

Figure 2.17a Unit Costs of Fire/Burn Injuries by Sex and Age Group, 2000

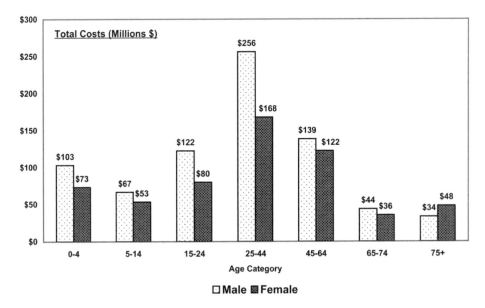

Figure 2.17b Total Medical Costs ($M) of Fire/Burn Injuries by Sex and Age Group, 2000

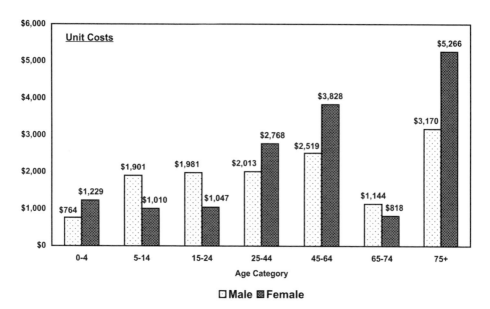

Figure 2.18a Unit Costs of Poisoning Injuries by Sex and Age Group, 2000

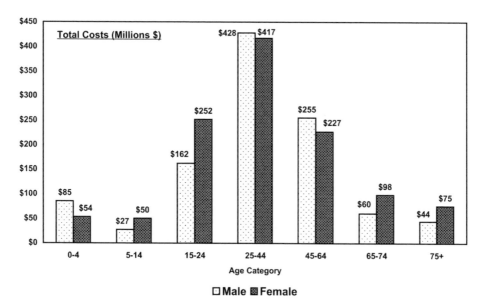

Figure 2.18b Total Medical Costs ($M) of Poisoning Injuries by Sex and Age Group, 2000

with the exception of persons aged 65 to 74 years. For men, unit medical costs range from $764 for those aged 0 to 4 years to $3,170 for those aged greater than 75 years. For women, unit medical costs range from $818 for those aged 65 to 74 years to $5,266 for those 75 years and older.

Drowning/Submersion

Fatal and nonfatal drownings, at $95 million, account for less than 1% of total injury-attributable medical costs. The majority of this total, or 96%, is represented by fatal (14%) and hospitalized (82%) injuries (Figure 2.12).

Figure 2.19 shows unit and total lifetime medical costs of drowning injuries by age and sex. The relatively high overall unit medical costs of drowning injuries are driven by the high unit medical costs of drownings that result in hospitalization. Drowning injuries among children aged 0 to 4 years, the age group with the highest incidence of drowning injuries, account for the highest percentage of total medical costs of drownings. In general, because males suffer more drowning injuries than females, their total medical costs of drownings are greater than those for same-aged females.

Firearm/Gunshot

Firearm/gunshot injuries account for less than 2% ($1.2 billion) of injury-attributable medical costs; however, they account for 8% ($85 million) of medical costs for fatal injuries (Table 2.2). As with drowning injuries, the majority (or 96%) of total medical costs of firearm/gunshot injuries are accounted for by fatal (7%) and

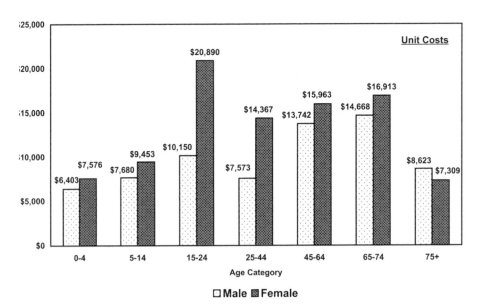

Figure 2.19a Unit Costs of Drowning/Submersion Injuries by Sex and Age Group, 2000

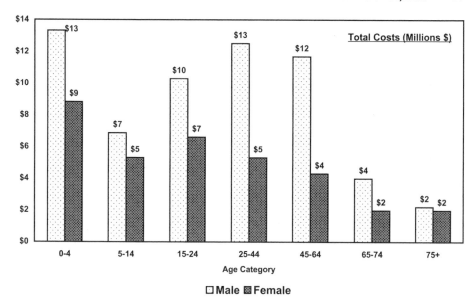

Figure 2.19b Total Medical Costs ($M) of Drowning/Submersion Injuries by Sex and Age Group, 2000

hospitalized (89%) injuries (Figure 2.12). This cost distribution is driven by both high unit medical cost estimates for more severe (i.e., fatal, hospitalized) firearm/gunshot injuries and the underlying incidence distribution; nearly 45% of all firearm/gunshot injuries result in death or hospitalization (Table 1.2).

Figure 2.20 shows unit and total lifetime medical costs of firearm/gunshot injuries by age and sex. Because males suffer more firearm/gunshot injuries than females at all ages, males' total medical costs are greater than those for females. For males aged 15 to 24 and 25 to 44 years, total medical costs of firearm/gunshot injuries are $453 million and $438 million, respectively. In contrast, total medical costs for females aged 15 to 24 and 25 to 44 years are only $37 million and $67 million, respectively.

Lifetime Medical Costs Data and Methods

The sections below present the data and methods for quantifying total medical costs for injuries. We calculate medical costs separately for (1) fatalities, (2) hospitalized injuries resulting in a live discharge, and (3) nonhospitalized injuries, that is, nonfatal injuries that do not require hospitalization, including injuries treated in an emergency department, an outpatient setting, or a doctor's office. Although not all data were from 2000, prior to conducting the analyses we converted all costs to year-2000 U.S. dollars using the relevant component of the Consumer Price Index (CPI) [U.S. Census Bureau 2003]. All future costs were converted to present value using a 3% discount rate.

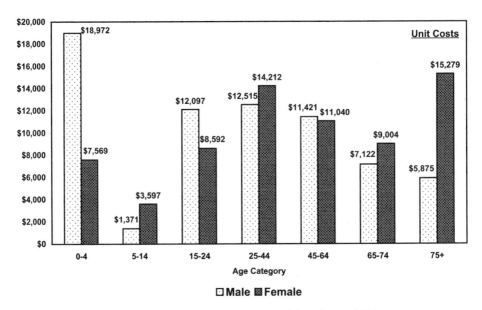

Figure 2.20a Unit Costs of Firearm Injuries by Sex and Age Group, 2000

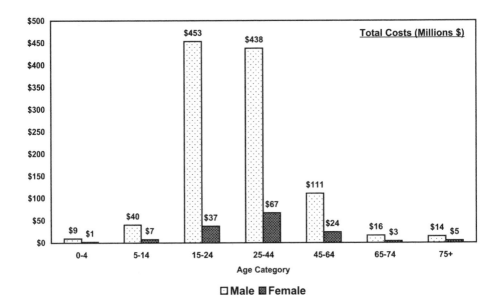

Figure 2.20b Total Medical Costs ($M) of Firearm Injuries by Sex and Age Group, 2000

Fatalities

We computed costs separately for 5 different places of death identified in the 2000 NVSS data: death on scene/death at home, death on arrival to the hospital, death at the emergency department, death at the hospital after inpatient admission, or death at a nursing home. The medical costs incurred, depending on place of death, might include coroner/medical examiner, medical transport, emergency department, inpatient hospital, and nursing home. Table 2.6 summarizes the costs included for each place of death.

All fatalities were assigned coroner/medical examiner costs of $530. This estimate was based on a dated survey of these officials [Edwards et al. 1981] and inflated to year-2000 dollars using the all-items component of the CPI [U.S. Census Bureau 2003]. Although these data are old, no newer costs are available, and no evidence suggests these modest costs have changed except due to inflation. Deaths on arrival to the hospital, in the ED, or after admission also receive the cost of one-way transport, which was based on average ambulance transport costs for injury victims found in the 1999 Medicare 5% sample.

For deaths on arrival or in the emergency department (ED), we also added average costs for injury fatalities in the ED by external cause grouping (homicide, suicide, motor vehicle, other unintentional) and age group (0 to 19, 20 and over) computed from 363 injury deaths in 1997 Nebraska, New Hampshire, and South Carolina ED discharge data. (These are the only states where we could readily get data with charges and discharge destination.) We first computed average charges using these data, and inflated the estimates to year-2000 dollars using the hospital care component of the CPI [U.S. Census Bureau 2003]. Because we were unable to get

Table 2.6 Data and Methods for Estimating Costs of Fatal Injuries

Location of Fatality	Cost Category	Description, Unit Cost (in 2000 US $)	Source of Data
At the scene/ at home	Coroner/ME (C/ME)	$530 (C/ME)	Edwards et al. (C/ME)
On arrival to hospital	Transport (T) + C/ME	$212 (T) + $530 (C/ME)	1999 Medicare 5% Sample (T), Edwards et al. (C/ME)
In the ED	T + C/ME + ED treatment (EDT)	$212 (T) + $530 (C/ME) + avg. costs for fatalities in the ED by external cause and age groupings (EDT)	1997 Nebraska, New Hampshire, and South Carolina ED discharge data (EDT)
In the hospital after admission	T + C/ME + fatal inpatient total (FIT)	$212 (T) + $530 (C/ME) + avg. costs for fatalities in the hospital by body region and nature of injury (FIT)	2000 HCUP-NIS for hospital facilities costs, 1996 and 1997 MarketScan® data for nonfacility costs (IT)
In the nursing home	C/ME + nonfatal inpatient total (NIT) + avg. costs for fatalities in nursing homes (NH)	$530 (C/ME) + avg. costs for nonfatal inpatient injuries by diagnosis (NIT) + $5545 (NH)	2000 HCUP-NIS for inpatient facilities costs (NIT), 1996 and 1997 MarketScan® data for nonfacility costs (NIT), 1999 National Nursing Home Survey (NH)

cost-to-charge ratios for these data, we adjusted average charges to costs by multiplying the charges by the ratio of the cost per nonfatal ED visit for injury (found in the MEPS) to the 3-state average charge for a nonfatal injury discharge.

For deaths in the hospital, we added the costs for an inpatient admission that resulted in a fatality to the transport and medical examiner/coroner costs. These costs were computed by body region and nature of injury using the Barell matrix and 10,889 raw cases in the HCUP-NIS file for those who died in the hospital. To all inpatient-facility cost estimates from HCUP-NIS, we added a cost for nonfacility services—such as professional services used while in the hospital, yet not included in the admissions billing (e.g., surgeon, anesthesia, physical therapy). These nonfacility costs were based on Medstat's 1996 and 1997 MarketScan® Commercial Claims and Encounters Database. This database contains an inpatient hospital admissions file, which has records summarizing each hospital admission, including total payments, facility payments, length of stay, and detailed diagnosis data. After removing non-fee-for-service claims and claims without a diagnosis of injury, we created a file with 19,247 inpatient injury admissions. Using these records, we calculate the mean ratio of total hospital costs to facilities costs according to body region and nature of the injury as presented in the Barell matrix. The ratios of total costs to facilities costs ranged from 1.03 to 1.39, with an overall average of 1.26. We multiplied the HCUP-NIS cost estimate for each admission by the ratio in the corresponding Barell diagnosis category to yield estimated total inpatient costs for each injury admission contained in the HCUP-NIS database. Costs were computed for nonfatal hospitalized injuries using this same approach (see following section).

For deaths in a nursing home, to the transport and coroner costs, we added (1) the HCUP-NIS/MarketScan® cost for an acute care hospitalization with live discharge for those with the same injury diagnosis plus (2) the average cost of nursing home care (565 raw cases) computed from the 1999 National Nursing Home Survey. Although we would have liked to use the average cost for those who died in the nursing home, the extremely small sample size prevented this analysis. To avoid double-counting costs for both hospital and nursing home fatalities, we subtracted from the total costs of fatalities in hospitals the costs of hospital care for those who died in the nursing home, since an inpatient stay with live discharge likely preceded the nursing home stay.

Hospitalized Injuries

We derive our estimates of direct costs for hospitalized injuries from HCUP-NIS data supplemented by Medstat's MarketScan® database for nonfacility fees, the Uniform Data System for Medical Rehabilitation [UDSMR], the MEPS, and hospital cost-to-charge ratios provided by the Agency for Healthcare Research and Quality (AHRQ). An overview of our approach is presented in Table 2.7. The details are provided in the following sections.

Total Inpatient Costs

We use HCUP-NIS data on inpatient facilities charges to compute inpatient facilities costs: each record in HCUP-NIS contains inpatient facilities charges for each in-

Table 2.7 Data and Methods for Estimating Costs of Nonfatal Injuries Requiring Hospitalization

Cost Category	Description, Unit Cost (in 2000 US $)	Source/Notes
Facilities component of inpatient stay	Average inpatient facility charges by strata (e.g., age, mechanism) multiplied by cost to charge ratios	2000 HCUP-NIS, Cost to Charge ratios from AHRQ
Nonfacilities component of inpatient stay	Estimated by comparing ratio of total costs to facilities costs by body region and nature of injury	1996 and 1997 MarketScan® data
Hospital readmission costs and probability of readmit	Probability of readmission and readmission costs by 3-digit ICD-9 codes	Estimated using 1997 CA, MD, and PA hospital discharge data
Hospital rehabilitation costs	Estimated for 14 diagnosis groups and 6 mechanisms.	Costs estimated using Prospective Payment System reimbursement amounts. All estimates reported in Miller et al. 2004
Nursing home (NH)	Costs added to HCUP/NIS discharges directly to NH. Costs estimated for hip-related fractures by age group and for all other injuries	1999 National Nursing Home Survey
Short-to-medium term (noninpatient) costs	Estimated as the ratio of inpatient to total costs in months 0 to 18 (on average) by select diagnosis groupings	1996–1999 MEPS
Costs beyond 18 months and up to 7 years	Estimated using ratios of total costs to 18 month costs by diagnosis/age group. Captures costs 7 years post injury	1979–1988 Detailed Claim Information (DCI) data from Worker's Compensation claims, Adjustment factor for youth from Miller et al. 2000
Costs beyond 7 years estimated for SCI and TBI	SCI: Ratio of lifetime costs to 7 year costs estimated from survey data TBI: 7+ year costs estimated at 75% of SCI costs	1986 survey data reported in Berkowitz et al. (1990)
Transport	50% of admissions assumed to have transport costs of $212	Mean cost estimated using 1999 Medicare ambulance claims with an injury E-code

jury, which we multiply by cost-to-charge ratios supplied by AHRQ. These ratios are hospital specific for 60% of the records in the HCUP-NIS file. For hospitals that did not have a ratio in the AHRQ data, we used a weighted group average ratio based on the hospital's state, ownership, urban/rural location, and number of beds, as recommended by AHRQ [Friedman 2002].

When computing direct costs of inpatient care, we exclude 20% of the HCUP-NIS injury-related records because they are missing either charges (some states do not provide this information) or, more rarely, length of stay. We also exclude 0.7% of remaining records because the per diem charge falls in the extreme tails of the distribution (less than $280, or greater than $20,920). We trimmed the distribution to produce robust means [Wainer 1976]. Using the approach described above for deaths in the hospital, we use Medstat's Marketscan® data to quantify nonfacility fees incurred during an inpatient admission for nonfatal hospitalized injuries.

Inpatient Readmission and Rehabilitation Costs

Nonacute care hospitals are not included in HCUP-NIS data. We estimate costs of readmission to nonacute care hospitals by using HCUP-NIS direct cost estimates of readmission to acute care hospitals.

We estimate costs of rehabilitation by using direct costs developed for 14 diagnosis groups in each of 6 mechanism groups by Miller et al. [2004]. These diagnosis and mechanism groups come from the recently instituted Prospective Payment System (PPS), which determines virtually all rehabilitation hospital payments, including professional fees. Miller et al. used PPS data on lengths of stay and cost per day to develop direct cost estimates of rehabilitative treatment. They use data from California, Maryland, and Pennsylvania hospital discharge systems to compute the probability of rehabilitation for each PPS diagnosis and mechanism group. We add to each HCUP-NIS/Marketscan direct cost estimate the product of the probability of rehabilitation and the direct cost estimate of rehabilitation developed by Miller et al., who estimate that roughly 5% of all hospitalized injuries require rehabilitation.

Nursing Home Costs

HCUP-NIS indicates injury admissions that were discharged directly to nursing homes. We quantify nursing home costs for these cases using the discharge file of the 1999 National Nursing Home Survey, a National Center for Health Statistics provider survey. The discharge file includes data on 540 nursing home discharges for injury: 13 traumatic brain injuries, 23 lower arm fractures or dislocations, 69 other upper-extremity/torso fractures, 345 hip-related fractures, 53 knee/lower-leg/foot injuries (fractures, dislocations, crushes, or amputations), and 37 other injuries. Each record includes information on diagnoses, total length of stay from admission to discharge (some admissions occurred prior to 1999), and total payments. Using these data, we have a relatively small sample size, so we quantify average nursing home costs for those with 2 types of injuries, hip-related fractures and all other injuries. For hip-related fractures we quantify average costs separately for 3 age groups, 0 to 64 years, 65 to 74, and 75 and older. We did not differentiate costs by age for those with non-hip-related injuries. All estimates were inflated to year-2000 dollars using the nursing home care component of the CPI [U.S. Census Bureau, 2003] and added to the HCUP-NIS/Marketscan® cost estimates in the corresponding injury category for those individuals discharged directly to a nursing home.

Short-to-Medium Term (Average 18-Month) Costs for Inpatient Admissions Not Discharged to a Nursing Home

It is almost always the case that injuries requiring a hospitalization will require additional outpatient treatment after discharge (e.g., for follow-up care). Treatment for the majority of these injuries will end after several weeks/months. However, treatment for more severe injuries will require extended treatment that may last a lifetime. In this section we describe our approach for quantifying short-to-medium term costs for injuries requiring inpatient admission that are not discharged to a nursing home. Longer term costs are described in the following section.

To develop estimates of short-to-medium term costs for injuries requiring an inpatient admission, we multiplied total inpatient costs for each record in HCUP-NIS/Marketscan® (as derived above) by the ratio of all costs in the first 18 months of injury, on average, (including costs for inpatient services, emergency-department visits, ambulatory care, prescription drugs, home-health care, vision aids, dental visits, and medical devices) to the total inpatient costs (including admissions and readmissions) for that kind of injury. We derive these ratios from 1996–1999 MEPS data. MEPS is a nationally representative survey of the civilian noninstitutionalized population that quantifies individuals' use of health services and corresponding medical expenditures for two consecutive years following enrollment. Prior to conducting the analyses, we used provider-specific data from the CPI [U.S. Census Bureau 2003] to inflate all medical expenditures to 2000. Because we limited our analyses to injuries with at least 12 months of follow-up, and because the MEPS data include costs for up to 24 months, our sample captures injuries with an average of 18 months post-injury treatment.

Although MEPS is the best source of available data for capturing nationally representative injury costs across treatment settings (e.g., hospitals, physicians office, pharmacy) even after pooling 4 years of data, the sample size for many injuries with low incidence rates is small. Therefore, to obtain robust direct-cost estimates, we collapsed injuries into broad categories prior to quantifying average costs. For each treatment location, we collapsed records into ICD diagnosis groupings based on the following guidelines (in priority order):

1. Groupings must be comprehensive, covering all injury diagnoses (including those for which MEPS lacks cases).
2. Groupings need to balance the goals of diagnosis-level detail and reasonable cell sizes. In some instances, we accepted cell samples as small as 5 in order to avoid combining radically dissimilar diagnoses into a single group.
3. The diagnoses in each group should be similar, either in nature of injury or in body region, if not in both.
4. Total injury costs (or the ratio of total injury costs to hospitalization costs for admitted injuries) should be similar in magnitude across diagnoses.

Using the MEPS data and the criteria detailed in the preceding paragraph, we calculated the average ratio of 18-month costs to total inpatient costs (including inpatient facility and nonfacility fees) for 15 injury-specific diagnosis groups, ranging in size from 5 to 61 unweighted cases. The ratios ranged from 1.02 to 2.13, with an overall average of 1.35. These ratios were then multiplied by the corresponding inpatient cost estimates detailed in the preceding section to arrive at 18-month costs for injuries requiring an inpatient admission.

Long-Term Costs

MEPS tracks medical costs for injuries for up to 24 months. Because we limited the MEPS analysis to those injuries with at least one year of follow-up, the typical injury has, on average, 18 months of follow-up costs in addition to the costs of the initial treatment. While this will capture the majority of costs for most injuries, some injuries will continue to require treatment and costs beyond 18 months.

Rice et al. [1989] estimated long-term medical costs from costs in the first 6 months using multipliers derived from longitudinal 1979 to 1988 Detailed Claim Information (DCI) data on 463,174 Worker's Compensation claims spread across 16 states. The DCI file was unique. Nothing similar in size, geographic spread, and duration has become available subsequently. Because occupational injury includes a full spectrum of causes (e.g., motor-vehicle crash, violence, fall), the DCI data by diagnosis presumably captured the medical spending pattern for an injury to a working-age adult with reasonable accuracy. Their applicability to childhood injuries was questionable. To address this concern, Miller, Romano, and Spicer [2000] analyzed the 30-month cost patterns (long-term costs were not available) of adult versus child injury using 1987 to 89 MarketScan® data on private health insurance claims. They found that the ratios of 30-month costs to initial hospitalization costs for children's episodes by diagnosis did not differ significantly from the comparable ratios for adults. By diagnosis, the ratios for children ranged from 95% to 105% of the ratios for adults. Thus, it is reasonable to apply the DCI estimates to childhood injury cases.

Noting that out-year costs are not inconsequential for some injuries, and for lack of a better alternative, we use ratios computed from the DCI expenditure patterns to adjust our 0 to 18 term cost estimates and arrive at estimates of the total medical costs (including long-term) associated with injuries. This method implicitly assumes that while treatment costs vary over time, the ratio of 18 month costs to total lifetime costs has remained constant between the time the DCI data were reported and 2000.

For those injury/age groups identified in MEPS as having costs in months 7 to 18 we multiply our 0- to 18-month cost estimates times the ratio of total costs to the costs in months 0 to 18 for the same injury/age group calculated using the DCI data. Although the DCI ratios vary by injury diagnosis, overall, they reveal that, using a 3% discount rate, 77% of the costs for admitted cases occur in months 0 to 18, and 88% of nonadmitted costs occur during this time period. These ratios suggest average multipliers of 1.30 and 1.14 for admitted and noninpatient-admitted cases respectively. For age groups that are not represented in the DCI data, we adjust the ratios as described in Miller, Romano, and Spicer [2000].

Long-Term Costs of Spinal Cord Injuries (SCI) and Traumatic Brain Injuries (TBI)

For several types of injuries, and especially for SCI and TBI, a substantial portion of the total medical costs will occur beyond 7 years of sustaining the injury. For spinal cord injuries, because data are available beyond 7 years, we compute the ratio of lifetime costs versus costs in years 0 to 7 and multiply the ratio by the estimates from the MEPS/DCI analysis to obtain total cost estimates. This ratio was generated from data collected by Berkowitz et al. [1990]. Berkowitz et al. surveyed a nationally representative sample of SCI survivors and their families in 1986, and collected data on 758 SCI victims, including those residing in institutions, those living at home, and those in independent living centers. The respondents (victims, families, or guardians) provided details of care payments during the past year, including payments for medical, hospital, prescription, vocational rehabilitation, durable medical equipment, environmental modification, personal assistant, and custodial care. These long-term cost estimates rely on the assumption that the now-dated Berkowitz data on medical costs by year post-injury mirror the expected lifetime costs for recent SCI victims.

Quantifying long-term costs for TBI is more problematic. Most TBI programs do not have longitudinal data on TBI costs. However, Miller et al. [2004] estimated inpatient rehabilitation costs by diagnosis group, including SCI and TBI, finding that among patients receiving rehabilitation, the cost per case for TBI averaged 75% of the cost for SCI. TBI patients, however, were far less likely to receive inpatient rehabilitation (6% versus 31%). We assumed the TBI patients who received inpatient rehabilitation would follow the same cost pattern more than 7 years post-injury as the SCI patients, but with costs equal to 75% of SCI levels. For very severe burns, amputations, and other non-SCI, non-TBI injuries requiring lifetime medical care, lack of available data will bias the lifetime cost estimates downwards.

Transport Costs

None of the data sets and analyses described include transportation costs. We assumed half of nonfatal injuries requiring a hospital admission also required a one-way trip via ambulance to the hospital. For each injury, we added half of the one-way average emergency transport costs based on 1999 average transport costs (inflated to 2000) for Medicare beneficiaries with an E code on an ambulance claim. There were 15,579 Medicare ambulance claims (including air ambulance) that were E coded, with an average cost of $212 in 2000. The estimated 50% transport rate may be conservative. The National Pediatric Trauma Registry, which captures admitted serious injuries, shows that from April 1, 1994, through November 5, 2001, 58.4% of 48,288 pediatric patients arrived by ambulance [NPTR Biannual Report, December 2001].

Nonhospitalized Injuries

We use MEPS data to quantify direct medical costs for injuries not requiring a hospitalization. MEPS participants with injury-related expenditures but without an inpatient admission were divided into 3 categories by primary treatment location:

1. Any emergency department utilization;
2. Any outpatient but no office-based or emergency room utilization; and
3. Any office-based utilization but no emergency room utilization.

Although the number of noninpatient admitted injuries in MEPS is much larger than the number of admitted injuries, even after pooling 4 years of data, the sample size for some injuries remains small. Therefore, we again pooled injuries into ICD groups using the guidelines presented above for hospitalized injuries. For ED visits, we arrived at 51 diagnosis groups, ranging in size from 5 to 419 unweighted cases.

For office-based visits, we arrived at 52 diagnosis groups, ranging in size from 5 to 867 unweighted cases. For outpatient clinic cases, we arrived at 7 diagnosis groups, ranging in size from 14 to 34 unweighted cases.

For each of the ICD groups and for each primary treatment location, we calculated mean 18-month medical costs by summing costs across all treatment locations of the same type (and including prescription drug costs) and dividing by the number of individuals who received treatment in that primary location type. We then applied these direct cost estimates to the incidence estimates in the corresponding diagnosis category and primary treatment location to quantify total injury costs for noninpatient admitted injuries without double-counting costs for individuals seen in multiple locations.

Transport Costs

We assumed nonfatal injuries not treated in the ED were not EMS-transported. For half of ED treated injuries, we added one-way average emergency transport costs of $212 (see Transport Costs section above). Table 2.8 summarizes the approach for quantifying costs for injuries not requiring a hospitalization.

Limitations

The cost estimates presented in this chapter are subject to several limitations. First, as noted in the chapter introduction, the estimates are almost entirely based on treatment costs for physical injuries. Many injuries, such as those resulting from sexual assaults, may result in mental health treatment but no treatment for a physical injury. These cases are unlikely to be identified as injury-related in the data, and would be excluded.

The net effect of excluding mental health costs associated with injuries is likely to be substantial. For example, based on a survey of mental health providers, Cohen and Miller [1998] estimated that 3.4 million physical and sexual assaults resulted in mental health treatment in 1998, often with no other medical treatment.

Table 2.8 Data and Methods for Estimating Costs of Nonfatal Injuries not Requiring Hospitalization

Cost Category	Description, Unit Cost (in 2000 US $)	Source/Notes
Medical costs	Estimated separately for (1) ED visits, (2) outpatient but no ED visit, and (3) office based visits only. Estimated for select ICD groupings	1996–1999 MEPS
Emergency transport	50% of ED visits assumed to have transport costs of $212. No costs for outpatient or office visits	Mean cost estimated using 1999 Medicare ambulance claims with an injury E-code

A second major limitation of our analysis was the requirement to use data from a multitude of sources. Although these were the best available data at the time of the analysis, some of the sources are old, others are based on nonrepresentative samples, and all are subject to reporting and measurement error. These factors may have incorporated significant bias into the cost estimates. Our approach was designed to minimize the potential bias. However, more current and nationally representative data would have been preferable.

An additional limitation of having to use multiple data sets was our inability to generate standard errors around the cost estimates. These costs are associated with great uncertainty, and readers are cautioned that the actual costs for any given injury category could be substantially higher or lower than the estimates reported here. Lastly, this chapter focuses specifically on medical costs and does not include other resource costs (e.g., for police services), productivity losses (described in the next chapter), or pain and suffering and other nonmonetary costs resulting from injuries.

Appendix 2.1 Unit Medical Costs by Age, Sex, and Treatment Location, 2000

	Fatal	Hospitalized	ED Treated	Outpatient	Doctor's Office	All Nonhospitalized†	Total
All	*$7,463*	*$18,042*	*$1,139*	*$891*	*$667*	*$944*	*$1,601*
0–4	7,840	12,589	986	771	770	920	1,088
5–14	9,476	13,461	1,066	894	608	884	1,028
15–24	4,555	20,165	1,148	967	607	977	1,462
25–44	4,609	18,130	1,195	891	645	969	1,460
45–64	6,747	19,215	1,168	876	632	898	1,620
65–74	10,995	19,117	1,180	938	830	979	2,465
75+	14,252	17,253	1,133	774	911	1,017	3,953
Male	*$6,576*	*$20,549*	*$1,153*	*$912*	*$722*	*$987*	*$1,673*
0–4	7,954	13,144	1,037	769	953	1,006	1,172
5–14	9,325	13,858	1,060	897	701	929	1,095
15–24	4,470	23,040	1,131	987	680	1,005	1,627
25–44	4,522	20,624	1,208	883	667	1,000	1,641
45–64	6,465	21,948	1,223	977	662	956	1,901
65–74	9,992	21,636	1,309	859	906	1,065	2,562
75+	12,880	19,656	1,207	875	972	1,083	3,964
Female	*$9,504*	*$15,708*	*$1,121*	*$867*	*$614*	*$894*	*$1,520*
0–4	7,682	11,829	917	773	375	787	958
5–14	9,746	12,755	1,075	891	507	824	939
15–24	4,869	14,825	1,176	936	530	940	1,233
25–44	4,892	13,931	1,178	901	622	932	1,239
45–64	7,510	15,964	1,113	794	608	845	1,363
65–74	12,881	17,503	1,087	1,007	764	909	2,388
75+	15,611	16,393	1,099	745	881	986	3,948

† This is a weighted average of ED treated, Outpatient, and Doctor's Office.

Appendix 2.2 Unit Medical Costs of Injuries by Detailed Mechanism, Sex, and Treatment Location, 2000

	Fatal	Hospitalized	ED Treated	Outpatient	Doctor's Office	Total
Total	*$7,463*	*$18,042*	*$1,139*	*$891*	*$667*	*$1,601*
MV occupant	7,238	29,168	1,230	718	1,178	2,777
Motorcyclist	9,121	35,853	1,319	981	589	4,325
Pedalcyclist	12,956	20,832	1,163	1,013	934	1,909
Pedestrian	9,717	38,022	1,224	813	633	6,844
MVT unspecified	6,881	24,846	—	1,022	905	1,656
Other transport	5,256	23,802	1,248	1,015	942	1,919
Fall	16,487	17,842	1,129	979	934	2,325
Struck by/against	8,969	17,198	1,040	963	716	1,033
Machinery	8,063	16,219	1,097	684	618	1,250
Firearm/gunshot	2,950	36,767	857	868	331	9,351
Cut/pierce	4,768	10,298	858	881	460	888
Poisoning	3,586	6,427	1,123	298	371	1,765
Fire/burn	16,801	18,818	1,594	821	248	1,736
Inhalation/suffocation	6,521	25,059	577	257	167	2,081
Drown/submersion	3,214	23,630	1,532	—	—	9,435
Bite/sting	10,526	6,586	758	849	361	563
Natural/environmental	6,875	16,819	1,561	564	714	1,040
Overexertion	7,116	12,405	1,559	934	699	1,368
Other specified	10,639	17,133	1,009	647	539	913
Unspecified	13,292	16,668	1,124	—	—	2,807
Male	*$6,576*	*$20,549*	*$1,153*	*$912*	*$722*	*$1,673*
MV occupant	6,882	32,553	1,361	683	1,760	3,506
Motorcyclist	8,934	36,151	1,312	1,063	589	4,270
Pedalcyclist	12,712	22,180	1,178	1,075	1,064	2,068
Pedestrian	9,359	42,054	1,299	1,192	—	8,923
MVT unspecified	6,502	27,801	—	1,051	943	2,037
Other transport	4,709	24,128	1,312	1,031	1,026	2,101
Fall	15,957	20,418	1,189	993	894	2,264
Struck by/against	8,782	18,022	1,049	1,005	822	1,125
Machinery	8,206	16,361	1,118	619	699	1,371
Firearm/gunshot	3,006	36,578	852	882	331	9,239
Cut/pierce	5,163	11,226	856	865	478	938
Poisoning	3,108	6,934	1,157	301	355	1,805
Fire/burn	16,049	19,687	1,595	898	225	2,054
Inhalation/suffocation	5,220	25,848	562	260	110	1,476
Drown/submersion	2,962	22,492	1,611	—	—	8,673
Bite/sting	9,747	6,718	772	858	368	623
Natural/environmental	6,040	17,309	1,578	848	833	1,637
Overexertion	6,907	12,360	1,433	920	728	1,247
Other specified	10,327	17,945	1,032	638	565	1,084
Unspecified	12,251	18,457	1,339			2,808
Female	*$9,504*	*$15,708*	*$1,121*	*$867*	*$614*	*$1,520*
MV occupant	7,918	25,062	1,120	732	873	2,181
Motorcyclist	10,891	33,505	1,369	908		4,838

continued

	Fatal	Hospitalized	ED Treated	Outpatient	Doctor's Office	Total
Pedalcyclist	14,570	15,758	1,120	754	650	1,479
Pedestrian	10,545	31,129	1,128	765	633	4,598
MVT unspecified	7,016	21,106		994	878	853
Other transport	7,781	23,113	1,172	933	791	2,648
Fall	17,119	16,401	1,074	967	963	2,374
Struck by/against	10,048	14,279	1,023	913	544	881
Machinery	4,735	14,913	979	716	373	774
Firearm/gunshot	2,613	38,254	892	601	—	10,291
Cut/pierce	3,689	8,047	860	923	432	802
Poisoning	4,590	6,072	1,080	296	381	1,729
Fire/burn	17,906	17,431	1,592	721	260	1,443
Inhalation/suffocation	9,174	24,143	593	255	636	4,145
Drown/submersion	4,044	25,826	1,398	—	—	11,177
Bite/sting	12,158	6,448	744	842	357	521
Natural/environmental	8,390	16,059	1,506	466	679	837
Overexertion	7,814	12,457	1,710	957	637	1,542
Other specified	11,868	15,961	971	656	524	776
Unspecified	14,487	14,848	737	—	—	2,805

* Motor-vehicle crashes from FARS

Appendix 2.3 Total Lifetime Medical Costs of Injuries by Detailed Mechanism, Sex, and Treatment Location 2000 ($M)

	Fatal	Hospitalized	ED Treated	Outpatient	Doctor's Office	Total
Total	*$1,113*	*$33,737*	*$31,804*	*$526*	*$13,068*	*$80,248*
MV occupant	242	5,327	3,470	12	419	9,470
Motorcyclist	26	823	222	3	35	1,109
Pedalcyclist	11	522	578	8	101	1,221
Pedestrian	59	1,146	180	1	12	1,399
MVT unspecified	4	383		30	412	828
Other transport	16	981	679	10	519	2,206
Fall	232	15,247	8,192	142	3,079	26,892
Struck by/against	12	1,474	6,199	117	3,226	11,028
Machinery	5	256	310	4	190	765
Firearm/gunshot	85	1,089	43	2	7	1,225
Cut/pierce	11	732	2,223	53	643	3,662
Poisoning	73	1,408	560	2	194	2,236
Fire/burn	66	461	736	15	66	1,345
Inhalation/suffocation	79	255	21	1	20	375
Drown/submersion	13	78	4	—	—	95
Bite/sting	1	179	911	42	740	1,873
Natural/environmental	11	257	50	3	579	900
Overexertion	0	527	5,423	42	1,164	7,155
Other specified	21	1,102	1,098	39	1,663	3,923
Unspecified	145	1,491	904	—	—	2,540
Male	*$683*	*$18,531*	*$17,976*	*$283*	*$6,972*	*$44,445*
MV occupant	151	3,259	1,747	3	215	5,376
Motorcyclist	23	736	195	1	35	991
Pedalcyclist	10	439	431	7	79	965
Pedestrian	40	799	107	0	—	947
MVT unspecified	1	239	0	15	179	435
Other transport	12	675	387	8	365	1,447
Fall	122	6,260	4,111	64	1,221	11,778
Struck by/against	10	1,204	3,915	66	2,298	7,493
Machinery	5	233	268	1	162	669
Firearm/gunshot	74	961	37	2	7	1,081
Cut/pierce	9	565	1,430	38	400	2,442
Poisoning	43	625	323	1	72	1,063
Fire/burn	37	297	399	10	21	764
Inhalation/suffocation	42	141	10	0	12	206
Drown/submersion	9	49	3	—	—	61
Bite/sting	1	93	473	19	262	848
Natural/environmental	6	161	38	1	153	359
Overexertion	0	279	2,716	25	831	3,851
Other specified	16	682	693	20	661	2,072
Unspecified	71	833	693	—	—	1,597

continued

	Fatal	Hospitalized	ED Treated	Outpatient	Doctor's Office	Total
Female	*$429*	*$15,206*	*$13,829*	*$243*	*$6,096*	*$35,803*
MV occupant	91	2,068	1,723	9	203	4,094
Motorcyclist	3	87	28	1	—	119
Pedal cyclist	2	83	148	1	22	255
Pedestrian	19	346	73	1	12	452
MVT unspecified	3	143		15	232	393
Other transport	4	306	292	1	155	759
Fall	110	8,988	4,081	77	1,858	15,114
Struck by/against	2	269	2,284	51	929	3,535
Machinery	0	23	42	3	28	96
Firearm/gunshot	11	127	6	0	—	144
Cut/pierce	2	167	793	15	243	1,221
Poisoning	30	783	237	1	122	1,173
Fire/burn	28	165	337	6	45	581
Inhalation/suffocation	37	114	11	0	8	169
Drown/submersion	4	29	1	—	—	34
Bite/sting	1	85	438	24	478	1,026
Natural/environmental	5	96	12	2	426	541
Overexertion	0	248	2,706	17	333	3,304
Other specified	5	420	405	19	1,002	1,851
Unspecified	73	658	211	—	—	943

Appendix 2.4 Unit Medical Costs of Injuries by Body Region and Treatment Location, 2000

Body Region	Fatal	Hospitalized	Nonhospitalized	Total
All	*$7,463*	*$18,040*	*$944*	*$1,601*
Traumatic brain injury	13,802	51,184	1,253	14,809
Other head/neck	6,678	10,614	800	1,049
Spinal cord injury	16,508	143,128	1,790	56,080
Vertebral column injury	12,696	11,600	1,003	1,199
Torso	8,187	13,442	805	1,591
Upper extremity	9,693	10,953	1,056	1,261
Lower extremity	17,996	17,815	1,099	2,085
Other/unspecified	7,559	11,434	739	811
System-wide	3,696	15,981	657	2,150

Appendix 2.5 Unit Medical Costs of Injuries by Nature of Injury and Treatment Location, 2000

Nature of Injury	Fatal	Hospitalized	ED treated	Outpatient	Doctor's Office	Non-hospitalized†	Total
Fracture	$15,119	$20,675	$1,537	$872	$1,147	$1,347	$3,907
Dislocation	$9,028	$14,254	$1,529	$1,615	$2,048	$1,876	$2,078
Sprain/strain	$9,033	$12,239	$1,412	$952	$600	$957	$1,017
Internal organ	$13,857	$36,683	$1,405	$616	$398	$1,236	$12,559
Open wound	$3,232	$9,481	$817	$843	$402	$740	$900
Amputation	$2,900	$16,999	$1,046	$675	$161	$897	$2,570
Blood vessel	$26,422	$29,258	$4,006	$589	$559	$1,128	$10,764
Superficial/contusion	$13,024	$9,533	$901	$876	$335	$702	$818
Crushing	$4,317	$13,015	$1,492	$1,040	$1,584	$1,512	$1,713
Burn	$6,619	$15,705	$1,781	$849	$198	$1,194	$1,689
Nerve	$14,720	$23,262	$1,887	$989	$731	$823	$1,854
Unspecified	$8,516	$7,145	$1,443	$1,003	$717	$1,201	$1,441
System-wide	$3,697	$9,333	$918	$406	$331	$683	$1,543

† This is a weighted average of ED treated, outpatient, and doctor's office.

Chapter 3

Lifetime Productivity Losses Due to Injuries

Injuries can result in both temporary and permanent disability. When this occurs, injury victims may lose part or all of their productivity potential. Losses in productivity due to injury may include lost wages and accompanying fringe benefits, and the lost ability to perform one's normal household responsibilities. For nonfatal injuries (i.e., hospitalized and nonhospitalized), productivity losses represent the value of goods and services not produced because of injury-related illness and disability. To the degree that injuries prevent or deter individuals from producing goods and services in the marketplace, the public sector, or the household, the value of these losses is a cost borne by society. Consistent with the human capital approach for quantifying the burden of injuries, estimates of nonfatal productivity losses involve applying average earnings to work-years lost and the value of housekeeping services to time lost in home production. Nonfatal injuries may result in both short-term productivity losses and in lifetime productivity losses, the latter includes the value of output lost by persons disabled in later years as a result of injury sustained in 2000.

We stratified nonfatal productivity losses into two categories: short-term losses, which represent lost wages and accompanying fringe benefits and household services occurring in the first 6 months after an injury, and long-term losses, which represent the respective wage and household loss occurring after 6 months from the time of the injury. Data availability drove the decision to use 6 months as the transition point between short-term and long-term disability.

Fatal productivity losses represent the value of goods and services never produced because of injury-related premature death. They are estimated by applying expected lifetime earnings by age and sex, to the 149,075 deaths from injury sustained in 2000 (Chapter 1), including an imputed value for lost household services.

For each injury category (i.e., fatal, hospitalized, nonhospitalized), productivity loss categories (i.e., wage plus fringe benefit loss, household service loss) are stratified by the following:

- Age and sex (for males and females in the following age categories: 0–4, 5–14, 15–24, 25–44, 45–64, 65–74, or 75 and older);
- Mechanism of injury (including motor vehicle/other road user, falls, struck by/ against, cut/pierce, fire/burn, poisoning, drowning/submersion, or firearm/ gunshot);
- Body region and severity of injury (based on the Barell Injury Diagnosis Matrix and the Abbreviated Injury Score [AIS]); and
- Nature of injury (including fracture, dislocation, sprain/strain, internal organ, open wound, amputation, blood vessel, superficial/contusion, crushing, burn, nerve, system-wide, or unspecified).

In addition, productivity losses for injuries that result from 8 major mechanisms are examined by age and sex. All future productivity losses are discounted at 3% to reflect present value, and all loss estimates are reported in year-2000 U.S. dollars. Specifics regarding the data and methods used to develop these productivity loss estimates are described at the end of the chapter. It should be noted that because men earn higher wages than women, even in the same job [Bureau of Labor Statistics 2001], for injuries with the same prevalence between men and women, the productivity loss estimates are greater for men. We view this as more of a shortcoming of the labor market than an inherent problem with the human capital approach. Regardless, this undervaluation of women's labor is reflected in the estimates that follow.

Total Lifetime Injury-Attributable Productivity Losses

Table 3.1 presents total productivity losses for injuries that occurred in 2000 by age and sex. Corresponding productivity-loss estimates per injury episode are presented in Appendix Table 3.1. Ultimately, injuries that occurred in 2000 will cause an estimated $326 billion in productivity losses: $142 billion for fatal injuries, $58.7 billion for hospitalized injuries, and $125.3 billion for nonhospitalized injuries. Figure 3.1 illustrates the distribution of total productivity losses by injury category (i.e., fatal or nonfatal), and treatment location for nonfatal injuries. Injury fatalities, which account for only 0.3% of all injuries in 2000 (Chapter 1), represent 44% of injury-attributable productivity losses. This highly disproportionate share can be attributed to the fact that injury victims who die prematurely lose 100% of their expected lifetime earnings. A similar, yet less profound, pattern is evident for hospitalized injuries, which are likely to cause disability both in the short- and long-term. Hospitalized injuries, which account for nearly 4% of all injuries, represent 18% of injury-attributable productivity losses. In contrast, nonhospitalized injuries, which account for 96% of all injuries, represent only 38% of injury-attributable productivity losses.

Short-term productivity losses (those losses occurring within the first 6 months following an injury) account for $9.2 billion (16%) of productivity losses for injuries

Table 3.1 Total Lifetime Productivity Losses for Injuries by Age and Sex, 2000 ($M)

| | Fatal | Hospitalized | | Nonhospitalized | | Total |
		Short-Term	Total	Short-Term	Total	
All	*$142,042*	*$9,179*	*$58,716*	*$58,040*	*$125,284*	*$326,042*
0–4	3,608	0	2,005	0	6,651	12,264
5–14	4,695	40	4,572	719	17,132	26,400
15–24	36,741	427	12,047	4,238	18,152	66,940
25–44	68,112	3,112	23,334	28,886	49,742	141,188
45–64	25,455	3,260	11,998	20,312	28,858	66,311
65–74	2,061	984	2,294	2,605	3,186	7,541
75+	1,369	1,357	2,466	1,280	1,564	5,399
Male	*$116,670*	*$5,396*	*$42,276*	*$32,068*	*$79,743*	*$238,688*
0–4	2,441	0	1,368	0	4,923	8,733
5–14	3,414	25	3,466	358	11,930	18,810
15–24	31,096	291	9,654	2,120	12,180	52,930
25–44	57,058	2,238	18,119	16,962	31,841	107,019
45–64	20,620	2,077	8,081	10,990	16,910	45,612
65–74	1,400	427	991	1,236	1,483	3,873
75+	641	338	596	402	474	1,712
Female	*$25,371*	*$3,784*	*$16,441*	*$25,973*	*$45,541*	*$87,353*
0–4	1,167	0	637	0	1,728	3,531
5–14	1,282	15	1,106	361	5,202	7,589
15–24	5,646	136	2,393	2,118	5,972	14,010
25–44	11,054	874	5,215	11,925	17,900	34,169
45–64	4,835	1,183	3,916	9,322	11,948	20,699
65–74	662	557	1,303	1,369	1,702	3,668
75+	727	1,019	1,870	878	1,090	3,687

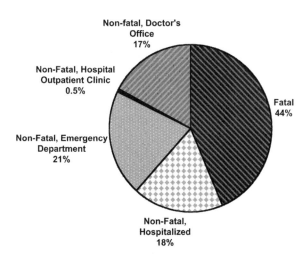

Non-fatal, Doctor's Office 17%

Non-Fatal, Hospital Outpatient Clinic 0.5%

Non-Fatal, Emergency Department 21%

Non-Fatal, Hospitalized 18%

Fatal 44%

Figure 3.1 Distribution of Total Productivity Losses of Injuries by Category and Treatment Location, 2000

requiring hospitalization and $58 billion (46%) of productivity losses for injuries requiring nonhospitalization (including emergency department visits, office-based visits, or hospital outpatient visits), (Table 3.1).

Injuries among males account for $238.7 billion, or 73%, of all productivity losses caused by injuries; injuries among females account for $87.4 billion. This differential does not necessarily represent different levels of injury severity between the two sexes; rather, it is partially driven by different levels of earning potentials. For example, an injury episode causes an average of $8,985 in total productivity losses for males, compared to an average of $3,707 in total productivity losses for females (Appendix Table 3.1).

Persons aged 25 to 44 years account for $141.2 billion, or 43%, of total productivity losses. Again, this difference can partially be explained by differences in earning potential across ages, where the average productivity loss per injury episode for this age group is $9,078 compared to an average productivity loss of $6,504 for all age groups combined (Appendix Table 3.1).

Table 3.2 further characterizes the productivity losses. It displays total wage (and accompanying fringe benefit) losses by age and sex, but excludes the productivity losses associated with lost household services. Injuries occurring in the United States in 2000 will ultimately cause an estimated $250.8 billion in wage losses, which represents 77% of total productivity losses. Figure 3.2 illustrates the distribution of wage losses of injuries by injury category (i.e., fatal or nonfatal), and treatment location for nonfatal injuries: $112.8 billion (45%) for fatal injuries, $43.6 billion (17%) for hospitalized injuries, and $94.3 billion (38%) for nonhospitalized injuries. Short-term wage losses account for $5.9 billion (13%) of total wage losses for injuries requiring hospitalization and $41.9 billion (44%) of total wage losses for injuries requiring nonhospitalization (Table 3.2).

Injuries among males account for $200.1 billion, or nearly 80% of all wage losses caused by injuries; injuries among females account for $50.6 billion. As with total productivity losses, the higher earning potential for males (average of $7,534 loss in wages per injury) compared to females (average of $2,148 loss in wages per injury) is partially responsible for this differential (Appendix Table 3.2). Given that household services are excluded in these estimates, earning potential becomes a greater determining factor in calculations.

Similar to the pattern for total productivity losses, persons aged 25 to 44 had the highest wage (plus fringe benefits) losses from injury ($113.7 billion). This represents 45% of total losses, while the injury episodes in this age group represent only 31% of the total incidence (Table 1.1). Again, this difference can be explained by loss per case differentials; the average wage and fringe benefit loss per injury episode for this age group is $7,312 as opposed to $5,002 for all age groups (Appendix Table 3.2).

Age and Sex Patterns

Figure 3.3 shows total lifetime productivity losses of injuries by age group and sex. For all age groups younger than 75, males account for a greater percentage of injury-attributable productivity losses than females. In fact, injury-attributable productivity losses for males aged 15 to 24 ($52.9 billion) and 25 to 44 years ($107 billion) are more than 3 times higher than injury-attributable productivity losses for females of the

Table 3.2 Wage (Plus Fringe Benefit) Losses for Injuries by Age and Sex, 2000 ($M)

| | Fatal | Hospitalized | | Nonhospitalized | | Total |
		Short-Term	Total	Short-Term	Total	
All	*$112,816*	*$5,868*	*$43,594*	*$41,944*	*$94,343*	*$250,753*
0–4	2,882	0	1,603	0	5,388	9,873
5–14	3,775	0	3,674	0	13,122	20,571
15–24	30,665	273	9,871	2,547	13,794	54,330
25–44	55,688	2,533	18,830	22,746	39,208	113,726
45–64	18,800	2,523	8,578	15,427	21,398	48,777
65–74	789	381	770	1,045	1,220	2,779
75+	217	159	269	180	212	698
Male	*$97,987*	*$4,289*	*$35,197*	*$26,523*	*$66,951*	*$200,135*
0–4	2,105	0	1,180	0	4,242	7,527
5–14	2,934	0	2,958	0	9,945	15,837
15–24	26,944	204	8,315	1,460	10,169	45,427
25–44	48,752	1,947	15,518	14,755	27,456	91,726
45–64	16,370	1,781	6,515	9,458	14,144	37,029
65–74	690	247	525	716	838	2,053
75+	191	110	187	133	157	535
Female	*$14,829*	*$1,580*	*$8,397*	*$15,422*	*$27,392*	*$50,618*
0–4	776	0	423	0	1,146	2,346
5–14	841	0	716	0	3,176	4,734
15–24	3,721	69	1,556	1,087	3,626	8,903
25–44	6,936	586	3,312	7,991	11,753	22,001
45–64	2,430	742	2,063	5,969	7,254	11,747
65–74	99	134	245	329	382	726
75+	26	49	81	46	55	163

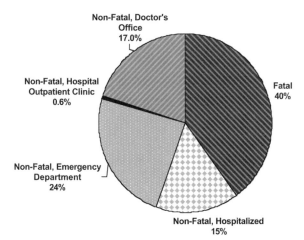

Figure 3.2 Distribution of Wage (Plus Fringe Benefit) Losses of Injuries by Category and Treatment Location, 2000

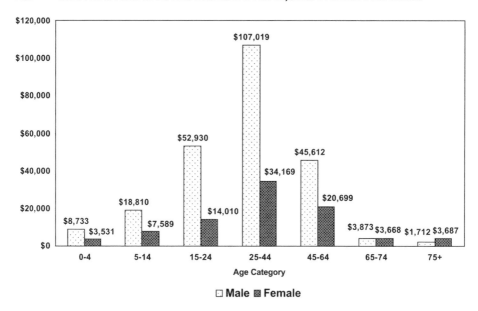

Figure 3.3 Total Productivity Losses of Injuries by Sex and Age Category, 2000 ($M)

same age. However, total productivity losses among females aged 75 years and older ($3.7 billion) are more than twice the productivity losses for injuries among same-aged males ($1.7 billion). Differentials in earning potential by age and sex (Appendix Table 3.2) partially explain these differences. For all groups, males had a higher average loss in productivity per injury (2% to 172% higher) compared to females. These same differences in earning potential by age and sex partially explain the total wage (and accompanying fringe benefit) losses by age and sex presented in Table 3.2 and Figure 3.4. Males had greater wage losses than females for all age groups.

For fatal injuries, total productivity losses for males are higher than those for females for all age groups younger than 75 (Table 3.1). This pattern is largely driven by the incidence of fatal injuries; for all age groups younger than 75, males accounted for a greater number of fatal injuries than females (Chapter 1), and the differential in average productivity loss per injury by age and sex (Appendix Table 3.2). At $112.8 billion, fatal injuries represent 45% of total wage (plus fringe benefit) losses (Table 3.2). Fatal injuries for males (almost $98 billion) result in wage losses that are 6.6 times higher than for females and, as Appendix Table 3.2 indicates, fatal wage losses per case are 2.9 times higher for males compared to females.

For hospitalized and nonhospitalized injuries, males account for a greater percentage of attributable productivity losses than do females for all age groups younger than 65 (Table 3.1). Hospitalized injuries caused $43.6 billion in wage (plus fringe benefits) losses in 2000 (Table 3.2). These losses represent 32% of total nonfatal wage losses. The wage (plus fringe benefits) loss was $23,314 per hospitalized injury and $1,961 per nonhospitalized injury (Appendix Table 3.2). Short-term wage (plus fringe benefits) losses represented only 13% of total wage losses for hospitalized cases as opposed to 44% for nonhospitalized cases.

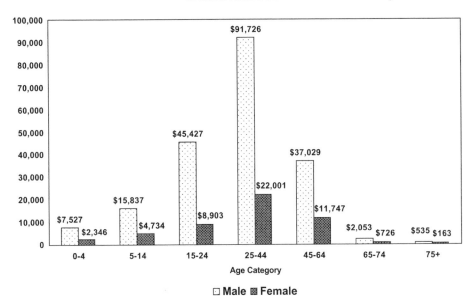

Figure 3.4 Wage (plus Fringe Benefit) Losses of Injuries by Age and Sex, 2000 ($M)

Total Productivity Losses by Mechanism

Table 3.3 presents total lifetime productivity losses of injuries by mechanism and sex. Corresponding productivity losses per injury are presented in Appendix Table 3.3. In 2000, motor-vehicle and other road-user injuries caused an estimated $75.1 billion loss in productivity. Excluding the category "Other," falls came second in terms of total productivity lost ($54 billion), followed by injuries in the category "struck by/against" ($37.1 billion). These 3 categories of injuries were responsible for 51% of total productivity losses. Figure 3.5 compares the distribution of productivity losses by mechanism and sex. Motor-vehicle- and other road-user–related injuries resulted in the highest productivity losses ($55.2 billion) for males, followed by falls and firearm injuries, which had similar losses ($31.8 billion). These 3 categories were responsible for 50% of total productivity losses in males. For females, falls resulted in the highest productivity losses ($22.2 billion), followed closely by motor-vehicle- and other road-user–related injuries ($19.9 billion) and then struck by/against injuries ($8.0 billion). These 3 categories of injuries were responsible for 57% of total productivity losses in females.

   Figure 3.6 shows the distribution of total productivity losses of fatal and nonfatal injuries, by mechanism. Motor-vehicle accidents and firearm/gunshot injuries account for 56% of the productivity losses of fatal injuries, 33% and 23%, respectively (Table 3.3). Nonfatal falls ($49.5 billion), struck by/against injuries ($35.7 billion), and motor-vehicle accidents ($28.5 billion) account for 62% of nonfatal injury-attributable productivity losses and 35% of total injury-attributable productivity losses. The most expensive types of injury per incident in terms of productivity losses were due to drowning ($0.52 million) and firearm/gunshot ($0.27 million) (Appendix Table 3.3). This is partly due to these injuries' tendency to result in death or long-term disability.

Table 3.3 Total Productivity Losses of Injuries by Mechanism and Sex, 2000 ($M)

| | Fatal | Hospitalized | | Nonhospitalized | | Total |
		Short-Term	Total	Short-Term	Total	
All	*$142,042*	*$9,179*	*$58,716*	*$58,040*	*$125,284*	*$326,042*
MV/other road user	46,609	1,857	15,499	7,395	13,021	75,130
Falls	4,524	4,315	18,481	13,373	31,024	54,028
Struck by/against	1,372	452	4,933	9,227	30,800	37,104
Cut/pierce	2,659	212	3,472	2,701	6,533	12,664
Fire/burn	2,985	68	713	929	2,504	6,202
Poisoning	22,760	332	409	483	538	23,707
Drowning/submersion	4,609	7	604	1	2	5,215
Firearm/gunshot	33,297	152	1,772	39	157	35,226
Other	23,228	1,785	12,834	23,893	40,705	76,767
Male	*$116,670*	*$5,396*	*$42,276*	*$32,068*	*$79,743*	*$238,688*
MV/other road user	36,514	1,257	11,362	3,774	7,337	55,214
Falls	3,621	2,056	11,277	6,108	16,926	31,824
Struck by/against	1,258	384	4,366	5,763	23,500	29,123
Cut/pierce	2,160	174	2,819	1,774	4,795	9,775
Fire/burn	2,122	44	517	392	1,439	4,078
Poisoning	17,792	169	225	277	302	18,319
Drowning/submersion	3,939	5	450	1	1	4,389
Firearm/gunshot	30,036	138	1,633	37	140	31,809
Other	19,227	1,167	9,627	13,942	25,303	54,157
Female	*$25,371*	*$3,784*	*$16,441*	*$25,973*	*$45,541*	*$87,353*
MV/other road user	10,095	599	4,137	3,621	5,684	19,916
Falls	903	2,260	7,203	7,264	14,098	22,204
Struck by/against	114	68	567	3,464	7,300	7,981
Cut/pierce	499	38	652	926	1,738	2,889
Fire/burn	862	24	196	538	1,066	2,124
Poisoning	4,968	162	184	206	236	5,388
Drowning/submersion	670	1	154	0	1	825
Firearm/gunshot	3,261	13	139	2	17	3,417
Other	4,000	618	3,208	9,951	15,402	22,610

Total Productivity Losses by Body Region, Nature, and Severity of Injury

Table 3.4 presents total lifetime productivity losses by body region. Corresponding productivity losses per injury episode are presented in Appendix Table 3.4. Traumatic brain injuries account for the highest loss in total productivity ($51.2 billion), followed by upper extremity injuries ($50.8 billion). Figure 3.7 presents the distribution of productivity losses among different body regions. Relative to incidence (Chapter 1), a disproportionate fraction of productivity losses are allocated to TBIs, SCIs, and system-wide injuries. These injuries, which accounted for 2.7%, 0.1%, and

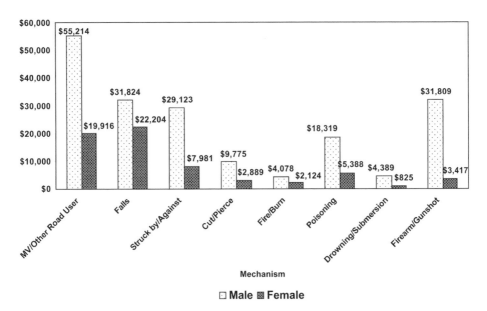

Figure 3.5 Total Productivity Losses of Injuries by Mechanism and Sex, 2000 ($M)

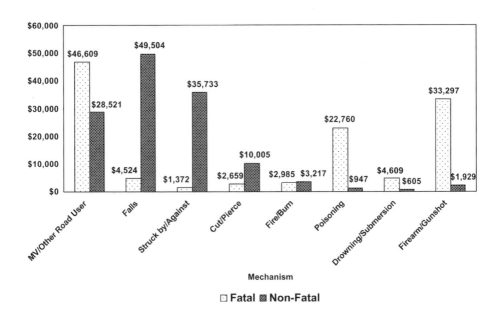

Figure 3.6 Total Productivity Losses of Fatal and Nonfatal Injuries by Mechanism, 2000 ($M)

Table 3.4 Total Productivity Losses of Injuries by Body Region, 2000 (Millions $)

| | | Hospitalized | | Nonhospitalized | | |
	Fatal	Short-Term	Total	Short-Term	Total	Total
All	*$142,042*	*$9,179*	*$58,716*	*$58,040*	*$125,284*	*$326,042*
Traum brain injury	38,550	594	10,063	693	2,598	51,212
Other head/neck	4,342	262	4,897	2,237	19,386	28,625
Spinal cord injury	554	77	2,891	57	227	3,673
Vert column injury	438	715	2,867	13,386	15,118	18,424
Torso	20,381	1,309	4,919	7,680	10,785	36,084
Upper extremity	677	1,281	11,953	12,239	38,208	50,837
Lower extremity	1,136	4,296	17,552	13,296	25,547	44,234
Other/unspecified	33,499	80	514	7,236	11,221	45,234
System-wide	42,465	565	3,060	1,218	2,194	47,719

5.9% of injury incidence, account for 15.7%, 1.1%, and 14.6% of injury-attributable productivity losses. In contrast, lower and upper extremities account for almost 50% of the incidence of injuries in 2000, and approximately 29% of the injury-attributable productivity losses. These differentials are due in part to the corresponding differences in productivity losses per fatal injury by body region. For example, SCIs and TBIs resulted in an average productivity loss of $135,713 and $38,126 per case, but $729,700 and $960,199 per fatal case. In contrast, the average productivity loss for a fatal injury to the lower extremity was $154,718 (compared to an average of $952,820 per fatal case for all body regions). Since productivity losses are based on age, gender, and the expected value of lifetime earnings, this suggests that victims of fatal injuries to the lower extremity were predominantly older.

Table 3.5 presents total productivity losses of injuries by nature of injury. Corresponding productivity losses per injury are presented in Appendix Table 3.5. Fractures ($71.9 billion), open wounds ($59.6 billion), and sprains/strains ($40.1 billion) account for more than 52% of the productivity losses of injuries. Figure 3.8 presents

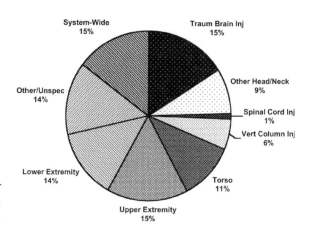

Figure 3.7 Distribution of Total Productivity Losses for Injuries by Body Region, 2000

Table 3.5 Total Productivity Losses of Injuries by Nature, 2000 (Millions $)

| | Fatal | Hospitalized | | Nonhospitalized | | Total |
		Short-Term	Total	Short-Term	Total	
All	*$142,042*	*$9,179*	*$58,716*	*$58,040*	*$125,284*	*$326,042*
Fracture	4,423	5,970	30,870	8,447	36,588	71,881
Dislocation	187	220	1,002	3,021	5,243	6,432
Sprain/strain	16	823	2,538	32,643	37,555	40,109
Internal organ	8,894	799	7,958	361	1,782	18,635
Open wound	32,185	285	6,419	4,201	21,028	59,632
Amputation	119	31	1,637	45	2,630	4,386
Blood vessel	1,688	8	269	5	9	1,966
Superficial/contusion	165	219	1,645	4,262	5,601	7,411
Crushing	765	22	224	351	915	1,904
Burn	1,078	74	836	857	2,860	4,774
Nerve	41	29	384	356	3,598	4,023
Unspecified	50,018	134	1,873	2,272	5,280	57,171
System-wide	42,465	565	3,060	1,218	2,194	47,719

the distribution of productivity losses among different natures of injury. Fractures and system-wide injuries, which accounted for 14% and 6% of all injuries in 2000, represent 22% and 15% of injury-attributable productivity losses. In contrast, sprains/strains and superficial/contusions, which represented 30% and 21% of all injuries in 2000, represent only 12% and 2% of injury-attributable productivity losses.

Table 3.6 indicates that, consistent with the underlying incidence distribution, the overwhelming majority (80.1%) of productivity losses associated with nonfatal injuries result from AIS 1 and 2 injury episodes, $79.2 billon and $68.2 billion, respectively. The most severe injury episodes (AIS 5) represent only 1.4% ($2.6 billion) of the total nonfatal productivity losses, despite having the highest productivity losses per injury, $99,806 per episode (Appendix Table 3.6).

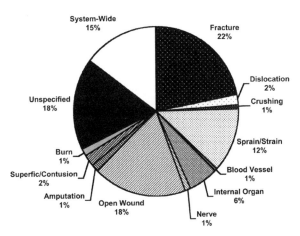

Figure 3.8 Distribution of Productivity Losses of Injuries by Nature, 2000

Table 3.6 Total Productivity Losses of Non-fatal Injuries by Major AIS Category, 2000 (Millions $)

| Injury Severity | Hospitalized | | Nonhospitalized | | Total |
	Short-Term	Total	Short-Term	Total	Total
All	*$9,179*	*$58,716*	*$58,040*	*$125,284*	*$184,000*
AIS-1	1,330	11,093	36,485	68,140	79,233
AIS-2	3,866	25,049	13,864	43,199	68,247
AIS-3	2,773	10,531	557	1,351	11,881
AIS-4	371	4,741	36	150	4,892
AIS-5	75	2,552	12	52	2,604
Unknown	765	4,750	7,087	12,393	17,143

Productivity Loss Patterns by Mechanism

The following section describes total lifetime productivity losses of injuries, separately for 8 major mechanisms. Productivity losses are stratified by age group and sex. Productivity losses per injury episode underlying the figures presented are detailed in Appendix Table 3.7.

Motor Vehicle/Other Road User

Slightly more than 23%, or $75 billion, of injury-attributable productivity losses result from motor vehicle accidents (Table 3.3). Fatal injuries account for 62% of this total. Figure 3.9 shows total productivity losses of motor-vehicle accidents by age group and sex. For both males and females, the biggest losses were observed in the 25 to 44 age group ($24.5 billion and $8.1 billion, respectively), followed by the 15 to 24 age group ($17.2 billion and $5.7 billion, respectively). This pattern reflects both the higher injury incidence and lifetime productivity potential for these 2 age groups. With the exception of the oldest victims (75 and over), males had higher productivity losses than females for all age groups. This gender pattern is mainly driven by the higher lifetime earning potential in males.

Falls

At 17%, or $54 billion, falls represent the second greatest percentage of injury-attributable productivity losses (Table 3.3). Nonhospitalized falls account for 57% of this total, making falls the leading mechanism of nonfatal productivity losses in 2000. Figure 3.10 shows total productivity losses of falls by sex and age group. For males, injury-attributable productivity losses for falls were highest among 25- to 44-year-olds ($10.9 billion). For females, injury-attributable productivity losses for falls were highest among 45- to 64-year-olds ($6.5 billion). This pattern does not reflect the underlying incidence of injury. For example, females aged 75 years and older suffered the most injury episodes from falls (Chapter 1), but not the largest productiv-

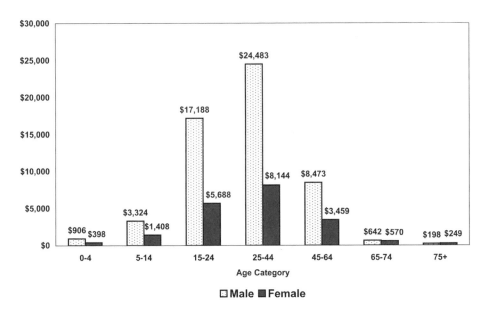

Figure 3.9 Total Productivity Losses of Motor-Vehicle–Related Injuries by Age and Sex, 2000 ($M)

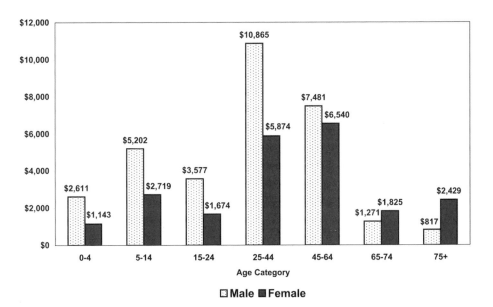

Figure 3.10 Total Productivity Losses of Fall-Related Injuries by Age and Sex, 2000 ($M)

ity losses. This differential can be partially explained by the higher lifetime productivity potential for younger people. With the exception of the elderly (65 years old and older), males had higher productivity losses than females.

Struck by/against

Injuries classified as struck by/against resulted in $37.1 billion of productivity losses in 2000 (Table 3.3). As Figure 3.11 indicates, for both males and females, the biggest losses were observed in the 25 to 44 age group ($10 billion and $2.6 billion, respectively), followed by the 15 to 24 age group ($7 billion and $2 billion, respectively). This pattern reflects both the higher injury incidence and lifetime productivity potential for these 2 groups. Males had higher productivity losses than females for all age categories except for those 75 years and older, where the loss for females was more than 5 times the loss for males.

Cut/Pierce

Injuries due to cuts or piercing by a sharp object accounted for $12.7 billion of productivity losses in 2000 (Table 3.3). Figure 3.12 shows that for both males and females, the biggest losses were observed in the 25 to 44 age group ($5.3 billion and $1.5 billion, respectively), followed by the 15 to 24 age group ($2 billion) for males and the 45 to 64 age group ($0.6 billion) for females. With the exception of the oldest victims (75 years old and older), males had higher productivity losses than females.

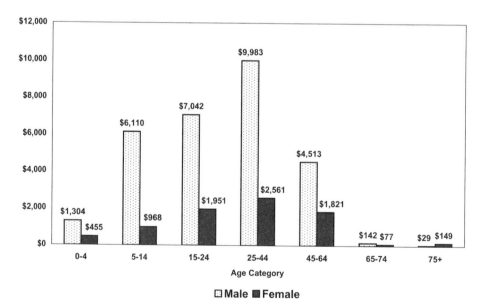

Figure 3.11 Total Productivity Losses of Struck by/against Injuries by Age and Sex, 2000 ($M)

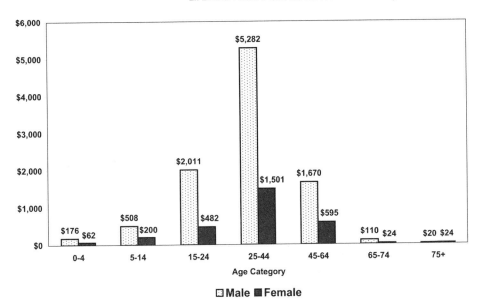

Figure 3.12 Total Productivity Losses of Cut/Pierce Injuries by Age and Sex, 2000 ($M)

Fire/Burns

In 2000, fires and burns caused $6.2 billion of productivity losses (Table 3.3). Figure 3.13 shows that productivity losses were the highest among males aged 25 to 44 years ($1.5 billion) and among females aged 45 to 64 years ($0.7 billion). With the exception of the oldest victims (65 years old and older), males had higher productivity losses than females.

Poisoning

In 2000, poisonings caused $23.7 billion of productivity losses (Table 3.3). Figure 3.14 shows that productivity losses, for both males and females, were the highest among 25- to 44-year-olds ($11.6 billion and $3.2 billion, respectively) and 45- to 64-year-olds ($4.3 billion and $1.4 billion, respectively). With the exception of the oldest victims (65 years and older), males had higher productivity losses than females.

Drowning/Submersion

Drownings caused $5.2 billion of productivity losses, 88% due to fatal drownings (Table 3.3). Figure 3.15 shows that for males, the biggest losses were observed in the 25 to 44 age group ($1.6 billion), followed by the 15 to 24 age group ($1.2 billion). For females, the biggest losses were observed in the 0 to 4 age group ($241 million), followed by the 25 to 44 age group ($207 million). With the exception of the oldest victims (75 years old and older), males had higher productivity losses than females.

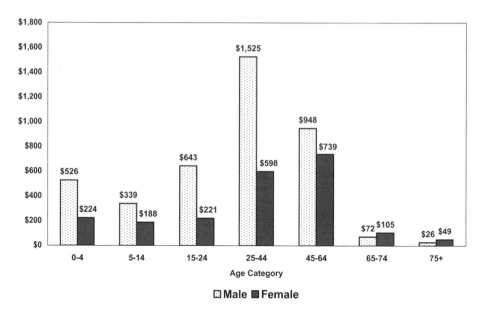

Figure 3.13 Total Productivity Losses of Fire/Burn Injuries by Age and Sex, 2000 ($M)

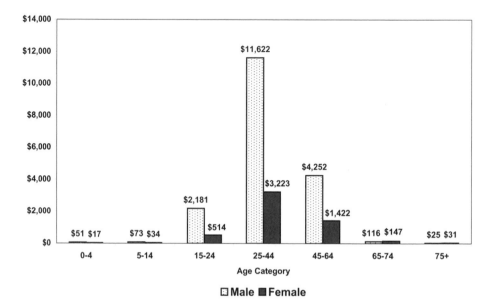

Figure 3.14 Total Productivity Losses of Poisoning Injuries by Age and Sex, 2000 ($M)

112

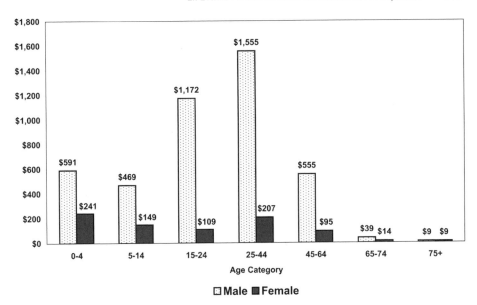

Figure 3.15 Total Productivity Losses of Drowning/Submersion Injuries by Age and Sex, 2000 ($M)

Firearm/Gunshot

Firearm-/gunshot-related injuries resulted in $35.2 billion in injury-attributable productivity losses in 2000, (Table 3.3). As shown in Figure 3.16, these losses were concentrated in three age groups: persons aged 25 to 44, 15 to 24, and 45 to 64. For males, productivity losses in these age groups were $15.4 billion, $10.7 billion, and $4.6 billion, respectively. For females, losses in these age groups were $1.8 billion, $0.8 billion, and $0.6 billion, respectively. For each age group, males had higher productivity losses than females.

Productivity Loss Data and Methods

The following section presents our approach to estimating the productivity losses due to fatal and nonfatal injuries.

Fatalities

Productivity losses for fatal injuries uses a nearly identical approach to that employed in the 1989 report [Rice et al., 1989]. For someone of a given sex and age who sustained a fatal injury, we summed the sex-specific probability of surviving to each subsequent year of age [Arias, 2002] times sex-specific expected earnings for someone in that age bracket (using 10 year age brackets) [as reported in Haddix et al. 2003]. Earnings, including salary and the value of fringe benefits, at future ages were adjusted upward to account for a historical 1% productivity growth rate [Haddix

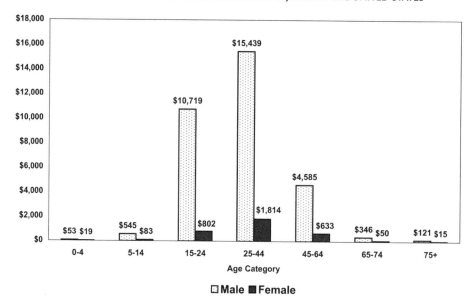

Figure 3.16 Total Productivity Losses of Firearm/Gunshot Injuries by Age and Sex, 2000 ($M)

et al. 2003] and then discounted to present value using the 3% discount rate used throughout this book.

Parallel calculations valued lost household work. Estimates of the value of household work are also included in Haddix et al. Historically, productivity growth in household production has been negligible, so we did not adjust for it. In all cases, we assume that the probability of surviving past the age of 102 is zero.

In equation form, lifetime earnings for someone of age a and sex b (Earn $_{a,b}$) is computed as

$$\text{Earn}_{a,b} = \sum_{k=a}^{102} \left[P_{a,b}(k) * Y_{k,b} \right] * \left(\frac{1+g}{1.03} \right)^{k-a}$$

where Earn equals lifetime earnings, $P_{a,b}(k)$ equals the probability that someone of age a and sex b will live until age k, $Y_{k,b}$ equals the average value of annual wages (plus fringe benefits) or of annual household production at age k for someone of gender b, g equals the productivity growth rate (0.01 for wages, 0.00 for household production), and .03 is the discount rate.

Nonfatal Injuries

For nonfatal injuries, productivity loss sums the value of wage and household work lost due to short-term disability in the acute recovery phase and of wage and household work lost due to permanent or long-term disability for the subset of injuries that cause lasting impairments that restrict work choices or preclude return to work. This section describes the methods used to estimate each component.

Short-Term Productivity Losses

We quantify temporary or short-term workloss for nonfatal injuries using the approach presented in Lawrence et al. [2000]. Lawrence et al. combined the probability of an injury resulting in lost workdays from 1987 to 1996 NHIS data with the mean work days lost (conditional on having missed at least 1 day) per injury estimated from the 1993 Annual Survey of Occupational Injury and Illness reported by the Bureau of Labor and Statistics (BLS). These data are sent to BLS by employers through a mandatory reporting system. Employers report work loss from date of occupational injury to the end of the calendar year for a sample of approximately 600,000 injury victims annually. All cases reported involve at least 1 day of work loss beyond the date of the injury. Moreover, if a worker still is out of work at the time the employer report is due to BLS, the report will undercount work days lost. On average, BLS work loss reports cover six months post injury. Lawrence et al. [2000] used a Weibull regression model to estimate the total duration of workloss for cases still open at the end of the survey reporting period. They combined these results with those of the closed cases to estimate average work loss, conditional on having missed at least 1 day of work. They then combined the BLS estimates with the pooled 1987 to 1996 NHIS data on probability of work loss to compute mean work loss including cases without work loss. Although BLS uses a detailed 2-column coding system (body part, nature of injury), we were able to map their codes to the ICD-9-CM codes for use in this analysis. We assigned the average work loss across all BLS cases to cases with ICD-9-CM diagnosis codes of "Other Unspecified" or "Other Specified." Averaged across all injuries, total estimated temporary work loss was 24.5 days per injury.

Although the BLS data are limited to injuries that occur on-the-job, a separate analysis of MEPS data (based on a much smaller sample) did not find that the duration of work loss differs by whether or not the injury occurred on the job. This suggests that the BLS-NHIS work loss estimates can credibly be applied to estimate work loss associated with non-work-related injuries.

Lawrence et al. [2000] did not differentiate work loss duration for admitted and nonadmitted injuries cases. We used MEPS data to quantify the increased duration associated with a given injury that requires a hospitalization. Although the MEPS injury sample is relatively small, thus not allowing for separate estimation by ICD or other strata, MEPS reveals that work loss is roughly 5 times longer for hospitalized injuries than for injuries not requiring a hospitalization. Using this ratio, we computed work loss durations for injuries separately for admitted and nonadmitted cases taking care to ensure that the weighted average across all injuries in the given strata (e.g., fractures) matched the result generated from the BLS-NHIS analysis. Averaged across all injuries, our estimated temporary work loss was 11.1 days per injury. This is slightly less than the estimate from MEPS, which was 13 days per injury. The highest temporary work loss was for AIS-3 injuries (52.5 days) and the lowest was for AIS-1 injuries (8.6 days).

To place a monetary value to temporary work loss, we multiplied the estimated days of work lost times the average wage and fringe benefit costs per day of work stratified by age group and sex from the Current Population Survey.

Following numerous other studies [including Lawrence et al. 2000; Miller, Romano & Spicer 2000; Zaloshnja et al. 2004], we estimated household workdays lost from wage workdays lost based on findings from the only nationally representative survey of injury victims that gathered data on household work losses following injury [S. Marquis, The RAND Corporation, Personal Communication, 1992]. That study showed that household work is lost on 90% of days that wage work is lost. Using this ratio and the value of household work reported in Haddix et al. [2003], we then imputed a value for household work lost. The estimates in Haddix et al. [2003] value household production lost using replacement cost. They start with national survey data on the average amount and nature of housework that people do by age group and sex, for example the hours that a 30- to 34-year-old woman spends on cooking and on cleaning. They value the cost of replacing these hours using data from the BLS on average wage rate by occupation (e.g., cooks, maids).

Long-Term Productivity Losses

To compute productivity loss due to permanent or long-term disability, we considered permanent total disability and permanent partial disability separately. For permanent total disability, we multiplied the present value of age- and sex-specific lifetime earnings and household production reported in Haddix et al. [2003] times the probability of permanent disability for each type of injury. For permanent partial disability, we multiplied the earnings estimate by the probability of permanent partial disability times an additional factor identifying the percentage of disability resulting from that type of injury. We then summed the results to compute the net productivity loss associated with permanent disability, including total and partial disability.

The probabilities of permanent and partial disability and the percent disabled by body part and nature of injury were reported in Miller et al. [1995] and Lawrence et al. [2000]. They used pooled multi-state Workers' Compensation data from the 1979 to 1988 DCI data base of the National Council on Compensation Insurance (NCCI) to compute these probabilities; DCI records the disability status for each sampled case. Application of these estimates to our analysis assumes that these probabilities are the same for injuries that do and do not occur on the job and that they have not changed significantly over time. It also assumes that the probability that an injury (e.g., a skull fracture) will cause someone to never do wage or household work again is the same for children, adults, and the elderly (the years of work lost obviously will vary with the age of onset) and that people will experience the same percentage reduction in household work ability that they experience in wage work ability.

We used the DCI probabilities in this study with the understanding that more recent data, although unavailable, would have been preferable. However, this data set remains the largest, most representative data set available for estimating disability probabilities by injury diagnosis. Averaged across all injuries, our estimated percentage of lifetime productivity potential lost due to permanent injury-related disability was 0.26% per injury. The highest percentage of lost lifetime productivity potential due to permanent injury-related disability was for AIS-5 injuries (8.1%) and the lowest was for AIS-1 injuries (0.12%).

To verify that the DCI data produce reasonable estimates, we conducted a literature review to compare our estimates to those estimated from other sources. Due to the paucity of data on this subject, we identified only a few sources with published disability estimates, and these were generally dated and limited to specific populations.

Traumatic Brain Injuries (TBI)

The Colorado TBI Registry obtained 4 years of annual follow-up data on a sample of all live TBI discharges in the state in 1996. Miller et al. [2004] analyzed findings on return to work for respondents retained for all 4 years. Thornhill et al. [2000] conducted 1-year follow-up interviews with a random sample of TBI discharges from Glasgow hospitals. Table 3.7 compares the DCI estimates of permanent disability with data from these studies and from a multi-trauma center study in Maryland that probed why people had not returned to work [MacKenzie et al. 1988] and a Seattle trauma center study with a control group [Dikmen et al. 1994].

The 5 sets of probabilities are similar for all hospital admissions. The probabilities from trauma center populations, as expected, are slightly above those for broader populations but none of these differences are statistically significant at the 90% confidence interval.

Other Injuries

Two other sources containing data on injury-related disability come from MacKenzie et al. [1988] and Butcher et al. [1996]. Both have fairly limited sample sizes and focus on specific types of injuries treated in trauma centers. Table 3.8 compares their results to the DCI estimates. As Table 3.8 shows, the DCI disability percentages are slightly higher than the trauma center percentages, although none are statistically different at the 90% confidence level.

Based on the limited information available, the DCI data suggest similar probabilities of permanent disability to the other studies of long-term work loss. Although dated and restricted to occupational injury, they have several advantages that out-

Table 3.7 Work-Related Disability and Return to Work of Hospitalized TBI Patients

	DCI*	CO	MD**		WA**	Glasgow
Hospitalized cases analyzed	2961	377	94		366	532
Did not return to work due to work-related disability, year 1						
All	17%	13%***	22%		21%	17%
AIS-5	37%		43%	GCS 3–8	60%	50%
AIS-3	14%		18%	GCS 9–12	31%	13%
AIS-1/2	12%		4%	GCS 13–15	7%	16%

Source: Computed from the DCI data, Miller et al. (2004), MacKenzie et al. (1988), Dikmen et al. (1994), and Thornhill et al. (2000).

* = sum of total and partial permanent disability probabilities

** = trauma center population

*** = the same percentage were unable to work in both year 1 and year 4

DCI = NCCI Detailed Claims Information data base, CO = Colorado, MD = Maryland, WA = Washington

Table 3.8 Work-Related Disability and Return to Work of Hospitalized Non-TBI Patients

	Spine		Extremities			
	AIS 4–5 SCI	AIS 3	Upper & Lower	Lower	Abdomen/ Thorax	All, Incl TBI, Other
Trauma center cases analyzed	8	18	76	312	37	262
DCI cases analyzed	30		59322	26812	5101	135055
Work-related disability MD; 3 trauma centers for						
lower extremity	52%	33%	21%	23%	5%	18%
DCI	65%	42%	27%	28%	7%	19%

Source: Computed from the DCI data, MacKenzie et al. (1988), and Butcher et al. (1996).

weigh their disadvantages. As a result of their large sample, they provide probabilities for a far wider range of specific diagnoses than all the disability studies in the literature combined. Despite its restriction to occupational injury, the sample also is more representative of the mix of injuries admitted to hospitals than the few studies in the literature, notably those which are restricted to patients triaged to trauma centers. The DCI data also are virtually the only source of information about permanent disability due to injuries not admitted to the hospital. The sample includes 318,885 medically treated, nonadmitted patients with valid lost-work claims in Workers' Compensation.

Limitations

The methods for estimating productivity losses have many limitations. Because women, the elderly, and children earn lower wages, the human capital approach applied in this chapter undervalues injuries to these groups. The approach also places lower values on the work of full-time homemakers than the work of people participating in the labor market, which further depresses the value placed on women's losses relative to men's losses. The approach places no value on a retiree's temporary or lasting loss of the ability to work and does not value temporary disability among children, as they have not yet entered the labor force. Discounting future work losses to present value means that the loss of a lifetime of work by a 2-year-old is equivalent to loss of a lifetime of work by a 43-year-old. Although the child loses many more years of work, those years are far in the future and heavily discounted. The productivity loss calculations are also based on a year 2000 life table, essentially assuming that life expectancy is constant over time. Moreover, the life expectancy for serious injury victims is shorter than for the average population, which may further bias the results. And, as noted, some of the estimates are computed using fairly dated data that are based on a working population. Finally, our estimates exclude productivity lost by people other than those injured as a result of an injury. These losses may include the time family, friends, and professionals spend caring for the injured, time spent investigating the injury, and worker retraining.

All of these limitations suggest that our results should be interpreted with caution. As new data become available this analysis should be updated to provide more precise estimates of the value of work and household production lost due to injuries.

Appendix 3.1 Productivity Losses per Injury Episode by Age and Sex, 2000

		Hospitalized		Nonhospitalized		
	Fatal	Short-Term	Total	Short-Term	Total	Total
Total	$952,820	$4,909	$31,402	$1,206	$2,604	$6,504
0–4	1,021,436	0	42,480	0	1,970	3,579
5–14	1,255,030	449	51,705	92	2,181	3,322
15–24	1,550,398	1,955	55,151	494	2,116	7,591
25–44	1,404,748	7,158	53,677	1,917	3,301	9,078
45–64	797,098	9,662	35,562	2,405	3,417	7,523
65–74	194,564	5,206	12,132	1,195	1,462	3,169
75+	50,532	2,446	4,447	491	600	1,693
Male	$1,122,908	$5,983	$46,879	$1,255	$3,120	$8,985
0–4	1,185,559	0	50,160	0	2,402	4,200
5–14	1,424,072	439	61,255	80	2,662	4,142
15–24	1,671,004	2,048	67,993	427	2,451	10,319
25–44	1,536,886	8,205	66,432	2,057	3,862	12,511
45–64	884,503	11,331	44,081	2,746	4,225	10,837
65–74	202,366	5,784	13,420	1,268	1,521	3,669
75+	47,588	2,313	4,081	480	566	1,717
Female	$561,626	$3,909	$16,983	$1,152	$2,020	$3,707
0–4	792,019	0	31,962	0	1,303	2,620
5–14	953,546	465	34,733	107	1,543	2,229
15–24	1,109,377	1,781	31,298	587	1,655	3,798
25–44	972,942	5,396	32,200	1,747	2,622	4,882
45–64	560,764	7,677	25,423	2,098	2,689	4,494
65–74	179,897	4,835	11,308	1,136	1,413	2,771
75+	53,449	2,494	4,578	496	616	1,682

Appendix 3.2 Wage (plus Fringe Benefit) Losses per Injury Episode by Age and Sex, 2000

| | Fatal | Hospitalized | | Nonhospitalized | | Total |
		Short-Term	Total	Short-Term	Total	
Total	*$756,773*	*$3,138*	*$23,314*	*$872*	*$1,961*	*$5,002*
0–4	815,870	0	33,958	0	1,596	2,881
5–14	1,009,084	0	41,544	0	1,671	2,589
15–24	1,293,996	1,249	45,188	297	1,608	6,161
25–44	1,148,514	5,826	43,316	1,509	2,602	7,312
45–64	588,698	7,478	25,427	1,827	2,534	5,534
65–74	74,481	2,016	4,071	479	560	1,168
75+	8,009	286	484	69	81	219
Male	*$943,086*	*$4,756*	*$39,030*	*$1,038*	*$2,619*	*$7,534*
0–4	1,022,510	0	43,243	0	2,070	3,621
5–14	1,223,982	0	52,265	0	2,219	3,487
15–24	1,447,901	1,436	58,557	294	2,046	8,856
25–44	1,313,159	7,138	56,896	1,790	3,330	10,723
45–64	702,184	9,715	35,538	2,363	3,534	8,798
65–74	99,739	3,351	7,115	734	859	1,945
75+	14,186	750	1,281	159	187	537
Female	*$328,263*	*$1,632*	*$8,674*	*$684*	*$1,215*	*$2,148*
0–4	527,023	0	21,243	0	864	1,741
5–14	625,818	0	22,489	0	942	1,390
15–24	731,208	902	20,355	301	1,005	2,413
25–44	610,477	3,617	20,451	1,171	1,722	3,143
45–64	281,844	4,816	13,395	1,343	1,633	2,551
65–74	26,999	1,162	2,122	273	317	548
75+	1,891	120	199	26	31	74

Appendix 3.3 Productivity Losses per Injury Episode by Mechanism and Sex, 2000

| | | Hospitalized | | Nonhospitalized | | |
	Fatal	Short-Term	Total	Short-Term	Total	Total
All	*$952,820*	*$4,909*	*$31,402*	*$1,206*	*$2,604*	*$6,504*
MV/other road user	993,452	5,850	48,829	1,276	2,247	12,197
Falls	321,932	5,049	21,625	1,250	2,900	4,671
Struck by/against	1,054,334	5,275	57,568	872	2,909	3,476
Cut/pierce	1,159,692	2,986	48,809	667	1,613	3,071
Fire/burn	760,971	2,770	29,067	1,246	3,357	8,009
Poisoning	1,123,346	1,514	1,868	469	523	18,705
Drowning/submersion	1,105,815	2,032	183,624	408	600	517,149
Firearm/gunshot	1,159,283	5,126	59,850	533	2,158	268,873
Other	846,486	6,748	48,511	1,579	2,691	4,979
Male	*$1,122,908*	*$5,983*	*$46,879*	*$1,255*	*$3,120*	*$8,985*
MV/other road user	1,132,395	6,418	58,004	1,253	2,436	17,041
Falls	473,551	6,705	36,783	1,250	3,463	6,118
Struck by/against	1,134,161	5,751	65,328	874	3,565	4,373
Cut/pierce	1,287,367	3,459	55,991	696	1,880	3,757
Fire/burn	909,633	2,891	34,313	1,104	4,058	10,963
Poisoning	1,296,728	1,881	2,495	570	623	31,108
Drowning/submersion	1,231,667	2,517	207,591	375	602	625,649
Firearm/gunshot	1,219,096	5,270	62,133	552	2,120	271,804
Other	1,109,419	7,858	64,809	1,832	3,325	6,965
Female	*$561,626*	*$3,909*	*$16,983*	*$1,152*	*$2,020*	*$3,707*
MV/other road user	688,073	4,933	34,041	1,301	2,042	6,821
Falls	140,913	4,123	13,145	1,250	2,426	3,488
Struck by/against	593,251	3,584	30,060	867	1,827	1,988
Cut/pierce	811,336	1,839	31,402	617	1,158	1,898
Fire/burn	542,703	2,576	20,701	1,374	2,723	5,278
Poisoning	759,588	1,257	1,430	379	435	7,940
Drowning/submersion	690,894	1,098	137,395	466	598	268,974
Firearm/gunshot	798,442	3,984	41,833	342	2,537	244,345
Other	395,711	5,327	27,646	1,324	2,049	2,958

Appendix 3.4 Productivity Losses per Injury Episode by Body Region, 2000

| | | Nonfatal | | | | |
| | | Hospitalized | | Nonhospitalized | | |
	Fatal	Short-Term	Total	Short-Term	Total	Total
All	*$952,820*	*$4,909*	*$31,402*	*$1,206*	*$2,604*	*$6,504*
Traum brain injury	960,199	3,817	64,681	604	2,264	38,126
Other head/neck	943,441	1,817	33,989	350	3,033	4,377
Spinal cord injury	729,700	7,446	280,262	3,542	14,223	135,713
Vertebral column injury	571,787	8,295	33,253	2,898	3,273	3,915
Torso	881,363	5,351	20,104	1,976	2,774	8,684
Upper extremity	764,679	4,653	43,418	938	2,928	3,816
Lower extremity	154,718	6,548	26,748	1,256	2,414	3,933
Other/unspecified	1,035,051	4,345	27,980	1,250	1,938	7,746
System-wide	1,086,477	2,025	10,963	464	835	16,205

Appendix 3.5 Productivity Losses per Injury Episode by Nature, 2000

| | | Hospitalized | | Nonhospitalized | | |
	Fatal	Short-Term	Total	Short-Term	Total	Total
All	*$952,820*	*$4,909*	*$31,402*	*$1,206*	*$2,604*	*$6,504*
Fracture	363,786	6,486	33,535	1,389	6,016	10,247
Dislocation	875,474	9,845	44,949	2,235	3,879	4,680
Sprain/strain	1,047,220	10,286	31,710	2,188	2,517	2,674
Internal organ	726,137	4,268	42,531	903	4,456	31,089
Open wound	1,151,156	1,835	41,348	481	2,406	6,682
Amputation	1,117,460	4,107	214,309	685	39,892	59,537
Blood vessel	807,820	1,376	45,567	359	596	86,465
Superficial/contusion	579,468	1,602	12,038	413	542	708
Crushing	1,048,056	7,249	72,662	1,921	5,007	10,203
Burn	1,033,375	2,764	31,419	1,122	3,744	6,031
Nerve	871,723	6,122	80,272	3,565	36,005	38,401
Unspecified	942,001	3,286	45,903	900	2,090	21,822
System-wide	1,086,477	2,025	10,963	464	835	16,205

Appendix 3.6 Productivity Losses per Nonfatal Injury Episode by Major AIS Catgeory, 2000

Injury Severity	Hospitalized		Nonhospitalized		Total
	Short-Term	Total	Short-Term	Total	
All	*$4,909*	*$31,402*	*$1,206*	*$2,604*	*$3,682*
AIS-1	3,401	28,370	1,114	2,081	2,391
AIS-2	6,506	42,162	1,659	5,168	7,624
AIS-3	5,793	21,998	1,867	4,523	15,285
AIS-4	4,707	60,126	665	2,802	36,939
AIS-5	5,308	180,176	1,002	4,352	99,806
Unknown	2,443	15,176	1,067	1,866	2,465

Chapter 4

Total Lifetime Costs of Injuries

The burden of injuries can be defined along several dimensions. Incidence (Chapter 1), medical spending (Chapter 2), and the value of lost productivity (Chapter 3) provide different views of how injuries affect individuals, the health care system, and the economy. This chapter quantifies the total lifetime costs of injuries that occurred in 2000, defined as the sum of medical spending and lost productivity due to morbidity and mortality. The magnitude of total costs is driven by several factors, including the initial incidence and severity of injury, the resultant period of physical impairment and disability, and, for fatal injuries, the number of life years lost. The contribution of each of these factors determines the allocation of total costs between medical spending and lost productivity. In addition to presenting total cost estimates stratified across many dimensions, this chapter demonstrates how the relative burden changes as the focus shifts between incidence, medical costs, lost productivity, and total costs.

As with previous chapters, cost estimates are divided into 3 mutually exclusive categories that reflect the severity of injury: (1) injuries resulting in death, including deaths occurring within and outside a healthcare setting; (2) injuries resulting in hospitalization with survival to discharge; and (3) injuries requiring medical attention without hospitalization. The latter category includes injuries requiring an emergency department visit, an office-based visit, or a hospital outpatient visit. Injuries that were not severe enough to require medical attention are not included in our calculations. We sum the medical and productivity costs of injuries across these mutually exclusive categories to quantify total lifetime costs.

For each injury category (i.e., fatal, hospitalized, nonhospitalized), total lifetime costs are stratified by the following dimensions:

- Age and sex (for males and females in the following age categories: 0–4, 5–14, 15–24, 25–44, 45–64, 65–74, or 75 and older);
- Mechanism of injury (including motor vehicle/other road user, falls, struck by/against, cut/pierce, fire/burn, poisoning, drowning/submersion, or firearm/gunshot);
- Body region (including traumatic brain injury, other head/neck, spinal cord injury, vertebral column injury, torso, upper extremity, lower extremity, other/unspecified, or system-wide based on the Barell Injury Diagnosis Matrix);
- Severity of injury (based on the Abbreviated Injury Score [AIS]; and
- Nature of injury (including fracture, dislocation, sprain/strain, internal organ, open wound, amputation, blood vessel, superficial/contusion, crushing, burn, nerve, system-wide, or unspecified).

In addition, the total lifetime costs of injuries that result from 8 major mechanisms are examined by age and sex. All future costs are discounted at 3% to reflect present value, and all loss estimates are reported in year-2000 U.S. dollars. Specifics regarding the data and methods used to develop these estimates are described in greater detail at the end of Chapters 1, 2, and 3.

Total Lifetime Costs of Injuries

Table 4.1 presents the total lifetime costs of injuries that occurred in 2000 by age and sex. The combined economic burden of medical treatment and lost productivity totals over $406 billion: $143 billion (or 35%) for fatal injuries, $92 billion (or 23%) for hospitalized injuries, and nearly $171 billion (or 42%) for nonhospitalized injuries.

Figure 4.1 shows the distribution of medical costs and productivity losses by injury category (i.e., fatal, hospitalized, nonhospitalized injuries). Previous studies have emphasized the high medical costs associated with injuries [Finkelstein et al., 2004]; however, the value of productivity losses associated with injuries, even for less severe injuries (i.e., nonhospitalized injuries), far exceeds the costs associated with medical treatment. The disparity between medical spending and the value of lost productivity is most pronounced for fatal injuries; 99% of the total costs of fatal injuries is attributable to lost productivity and 1% is attributable to medical treatment. In comparison, 64% and 73% of the total costs of hospitalized and nonhospitalized injuries, respectively, are attributable to lost productivity, and 36% and 27% of the total costs of hospitalized and nonhospitalized injuries, respectively, are attributable to medical treatment.

Figure 4.2 compares the burden of injuries, by injury category, across the following dimensions: incidence, medical costs, productivity losses, and total costs. Nonhospitalized injuries, which represent 96% of injuries, account for only 42% of the total costs of injuries. Conversely, fatal injuries, which represent less than 1% of injuries, account for 35% of the total costs of injuries; and hospitalized injuries, which represent less than 4% of injuries, account for 23% of the total costs of injuries. Although the percentages of total costs accounted for by fatal and hospitalized injuries are high relative to their incidence, the explanation for their disproportionately high

Table 4.1 Total Lifetime Costs of Injuries by Age and Sex, 2000 ($M)

	Fatal	Hospitalized	Nonhospitalized	Total
All	*$143,154*	*$92,453*	*$170,682*	*$406,289*
0–4	3,635	2,599	9,757	15,992
5–14	4,731	5,763	24,076	34,569
15–24	36,849	16,452	26,534	79,835
25–44	68,335	31,215	64,341	163,892
45–64	25,671	18,480	36,438	80,589
65–74	2,178	5,909	5,319	13,406
75+	1,755	12,035	4,217	18,007
Male	*$117,353*	*$60,806*	*$104,973*	*$283,133*
0–4	2,457	1,727	6,986	11,170
5–14	3,436	4,251	16,096	23,783
15–24	31,179	12,926	17,172	61,276
25–44	57,226	23,744	40,082	121,052
45–64	20,771	12,105	20,735	53,611
65–74	1,469	2,588	2,521	6,578
75+	815	3,467	1,381	5,663
Female	*$25,801*	*$31,647*	*$65,709*	*$123,156*
0–4	1,178	872	2,772	4,822
5–14	1,295	1,512	7,979	10,786
15–24	5,670	3,526	9,362	18,559
25–44	11,109	7,472	24,259	42,840
45–64	4,900	6,376	15,703	26,978
65–74	709	3,321	2,798	6,828
75+	940	8,568	2,835	12,343

cost differs. Fatal injuries are responsible for 44% of the total costs of lost productivity and 1% of the total costs of medical treatment. Conversely, hospitalized injuries account for 18% of the total costs of lost productivity and 42% of the total costs of medical treatment (Figure 4.2). In other words, the high cost of fatal injuries is largely explained by relatively high productivity losses, while the high cost of hospitalized injuries is largely explained by relatively high medical spending.

Age and Sex Patterns

The distribution of total costs of injuries across each age group closely resembles the distribution of the U.S. population, with a few exceptions. Persons aged 25 to 44 years represent 30% of the U.S. population and 40% ($164 billion) of the total costs of injuries (Table 4.1). Conversely, persons aged 5 to 14 years represent 15% of the U.S. population and 9% ($34.6 billion) of the total costs of injuries. The disproportionately high total costs of injuries among persons aged 25 to 44 years and the disproportionately low total costs of injuries among persons aged 5 to 14 years are driven by high and low productivity losses, respectively.

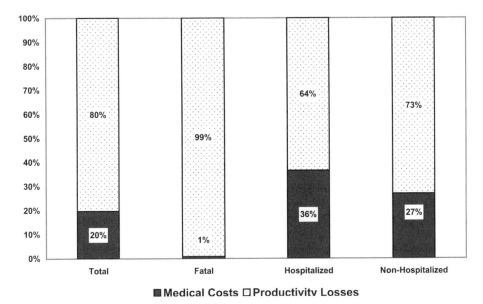

Figure 4.1 Distribution of Medical Costs and Productivity Losses by Injury Category, 2000

Figure 4.3 shows the percentage of total costs attributable to medical spending and productivity losses, by age. Lost productivity accounts for the highest percentage of total costs among the working age population: for example, lost productivity accounts for 86% of the total costs of injuries for persons aged 25 to 44 years. Because the elderly and children are less likely to be employed, their productivity losses as a percentage of total costs are low relative to middle-age adults: for example, lost productivity accounts for only 30% of the total costs of injuries for persons aged 75 years and greater. Unlike the elderly, however, children—if they die prematurely—will forgo a lifetime of wages; therefore, *fatal* injuries to children are associated with

Incidence

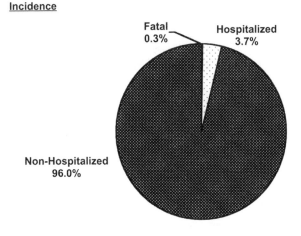

Figure 4.2a Distribution of Injury Incidence by Injury Category

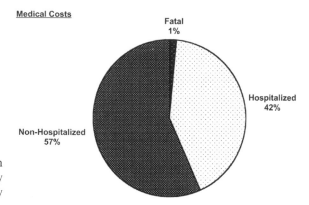

Figure 4.2b Distribution
of Medical Costs by
Injury Category

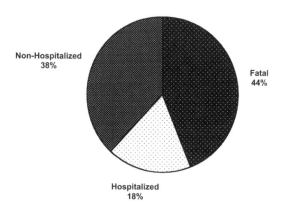

Figure 4.2c Distribution
of Productivity Losses by
Injury Category

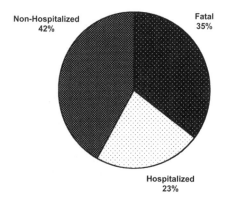

Figure 4.2d Distribution
of Total Costs by
Injury Category

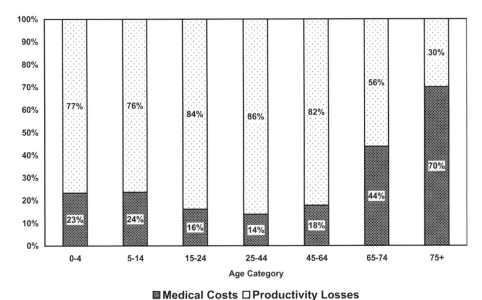

Figure 4.3 Distribution of Medical Costs and Productivity Losses by Age, 2000

very high productivity losses. As a result, lost productivity as a percentage of total costs for children, while low relative to working age adults, is still much higher than that for the elderly: for example, lost productivity accounts for 77% of the total costs of injuries for persons aged 0 to 4 years.

Males, who represent less than 50% of the U.S. population, account for approximately 70% ($283 billion) of the total costs of injuries (Table 4.1). This cost disparity is due, in part, to a slightly higher incidence of overall injuries and a substantially higher incidence of fatal injuries: males account for 53% of all injuries and 70% of fatal injuries (Chapter 1). Additionally, because males have a higher average wage than females, the value of lost productivity resulting from any given injury is higher for males than for females. We view this bias as a shortcoming of the labor market which leads to a shortcoming of the human capital approach for quantifying costs of illness/injury.

Figure 4.4 shows the total lifetime costs of injuries by age and sex. While males account for a higher percentage of total costs than females for all age groups younger than 65 years, females account for nearly 51% of the total costs of injuries for persons aged 65 to 74 years and nearly 69% of the total cost of injuries for persons age 75 years and older. Following age 65, several factors serve to increase the relative proportion of total costs accounted for by females: because elderly males and females leave the workforce, the lost productivity resulting from any given injury is roughly equal; additionally, elderly females account for a higher percentage of the U.S. population than elderly males and, therefore, a higher percentage of injury incidence (Chapter 1).

Figure 4.5 compares the total costs of fatal, hospitalized, and nonhospitalized injuries by age and sex. Across all age groups, males account for 82% ($117 billion) of

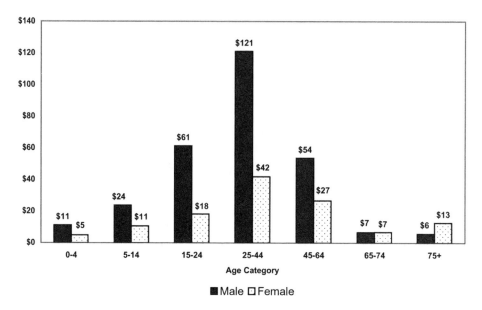

Figure 4.4 Total Lifetime Costs of Injuries by Age and Sex, 2000 ($B)

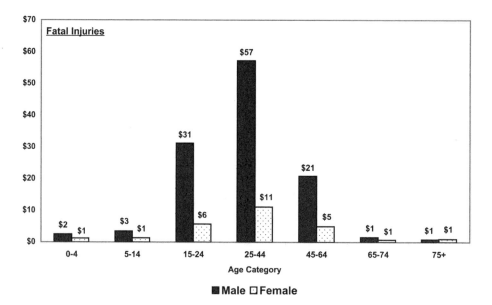

Figure 4.5a Total Costs of Fatal Injuries by Age and Sex, 2000 ($B)

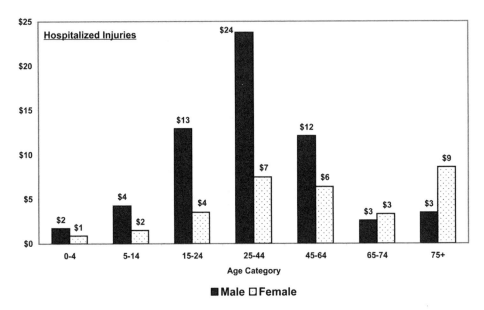

Figure 4.5b Total Costs of Hospitalized Injuries by Age and Sex, 2000 ($B)

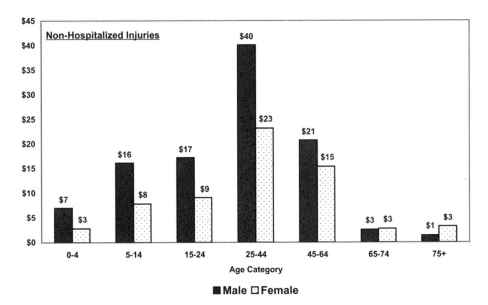

Figure 4.5c Total Costs of Nonhospitalized Injuries by Age and Sex, 2000 ($B)

the total costs of fatal injuries, 66% ($61 billion) of the total costs of hospitalized injuries, and nearly 62% ($105 billion) of the total costs of nonhospitalized injuries (Table 4.1). Males aged 25 to 44 years, who represent roughly 15% of the U.S. population, account for 40%, 26%, and 23% of the total costs of fatal, hospitalized, and nonhospitalized injuries, respectively.

Total Lifetime Costs of Injuries by Mechanism

Table 4.2 presents the total lifetime costs of injuries by mechanism and sex. Motor-vehicle and fall injuries account for 22% ($89 billion) and 20% ($81 billion) of the total costs of injuries; struck by/against and firearm/gunshot injuries account for 12% ($48 billion) and 9% ($36 billion) of the total costs of injuries.

Table 4.2 Total Costs of Injuries by Mechanism and Sex, 2000 ($M)

	Fatal	Hospitalized	Nonhospitalized	Total
All	*$143,154*	*$92,453*	*$170,682*	*$406,289*
MV/other road user	46,952	23,700	18,505	89,156
Fall	4,756	33,728	42,436	80,920
Struck by/against	1,383	6,407	40,342	48,132
Cut/pierce	2,670	4,204	9,452	16,326
Fire/burn	3,051	1,174	3,322	7,546
Poisoning	22,833	1,817	1,294	25,944
Drowning/submersion	4,622	682	6	5,310
Firearm/gunshot	33,381	2,861	209	36,451
Other	23,505	17,881	55,116	96,505
Male	*$117,353*	*$60,806*	*$104,973*	*$283,133*
MV/other road user	36,737	16,835	10,353	63,927
Fall	3,743	17,537	22,322	43,602
Struck by/against	1,267	5,570	29,778	36,617
Cut/pierce	2,169	3,385	6,663	12,217
Fire/burn	2,160	814	1,869	4,842
Poisoning	17,834	849	698	19,382
Drowning/submersion	3,948	498	4	4,450
Firearm/gunshot	30,109	2,594	186	32,890
Other	19,385	12,724	33,101	65,207
Female	*$25,800*	*$31,647*	*$65,709*	*$123,156*
MV/other road user	10,215	6,864	8,153	25,229
Fall	1,012	16,191	20,115	37,318
Struck by/against	116	836	10,564	11,516
Cut/pierce	501	820	2,789	4,109
Fire/burn	891	360	1,453	2,704
Poisoning	4,999	968	596	6,562
Drowning/submersion	674	183	2	859
Firearm/gunshot	3,272	267	22	3,561
Other	4,120	5,158	22,015	31,298

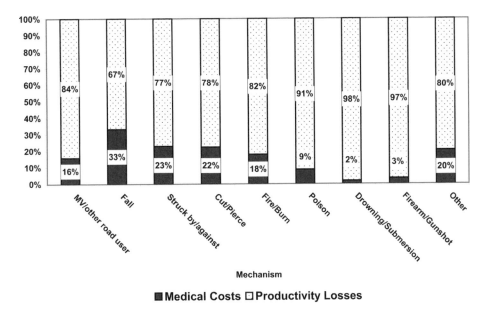

■ Medical Costs □ Productivity Losses

Figure 4.6 Distribution of Medical Costs and Productivity Losses, by Mechanism

Figure 4.6 shows the distribution of total costs (i.e., medical costs, productivity losses), by mechanism. Regardless of the mechanism, the value of lost productivity accounts for at least 67% of the total costs of injuries; however, the relative distribution of total costs between lost productivity and medical spending differs across mechanisms.

Mechanisms that have high fatality rates or high incidence rates among working-age populations have a relatively higher percentage of total costs attributable to lost productivity. This results because work loss due to morbidity or mortality is likely to be large, and, for fatal injuries, medical costs are relatively small. For example, due to their high fatality rate, 97% of the total costs of firearm/gunshot injuries are attributable to lost productivity and only 3% are attributable to medical spending (see Chapter 5). In contrast, mechanisms that have a high incidence rate among the elderly have a lower percentage of total costs attributable to lost productivity: for example, 67% of the total costs of fall injuries are attributable to lost productivity and 33% are attributable to medical spending. This results because fall injuries are more likely to occur among elderly populations who earn lower wages and are less likely to be employed, and whose injuries are generally more expensive to treat.

Figure 4.7 shows the total lifetime costs of injuries by mechanism and sex. Males account for nearly 70% of the total costs of injuries regardless of mechanism, accounting for at least 75% of the total costs of firearm/gunshot (90%, or $33 billion), drowning/submersion (84%, or $4 billion), struck by/against (76%, or $37 billion), cut/pierce (75%, or $12 billion), and poisoning injuries (75%, or $19 billion) (Table 4.2). Moreover, as shown in Figure 4.8, this pattern of higher costs among males holds for fatal, hospitalized, and nonhospitalized injuries. Higher costs among

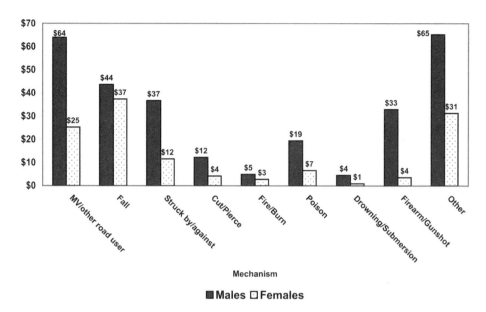

Figure 4.7 Total Lifetime Costs of Injuries by Mechanism and Sex, 2000 ($B)

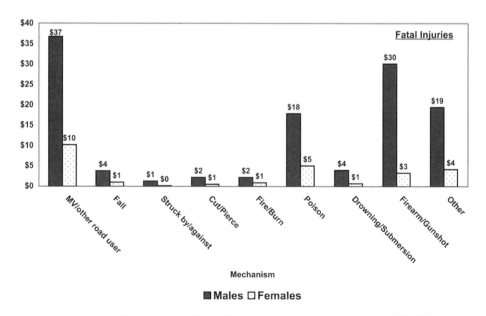

Figure 4.8a Total Lifetime Costs of Fatal Injuries by Mechanism and Sex, 2000 ($B)

134

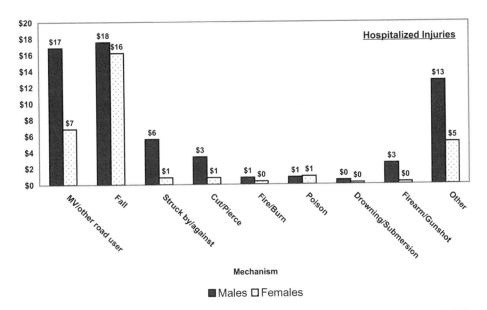

Figure 4.8b Total Lifetime Costs of Hospitalized Injuries by Mechanism and Sex, 2000 ($B)

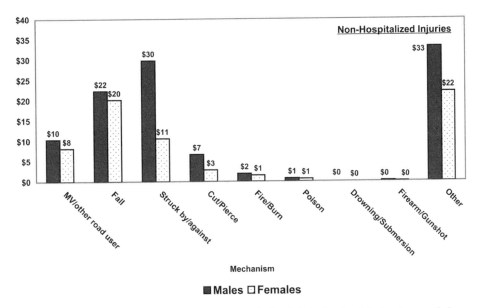

Figure 4.8c Total Lifetime Costs of Nonhospitalized Injuries by Mechanism and Sex, 2000 ($B)

males are largely driven by higher incidence rates, especially for fatal injuries, and also by greater productivity losses due to their higher wage rates.

Figure 4.8 also demonstrates the differential burden of total costs when stratified by injury category (i.e., fatal, hospitalized, nonhospitalized): the total costs of fatal injuries are largely attributable to motor-vehicle (33%), poisoning (16%), and firearm/gunshot (23%) injuries; the total costs of hospitalized injuries are largely attributable to motor-vehicle (26%) and fall (36%) injuries; and the total costs of nonhospitalized injuries are largely attributable to fall (25%) and struck by/against (24%) injuries. The differences in total costs are largely driven by where each mechanism of injury is most likely to be treated. For example, motor-vehicle injuries are more likely to result in fatalities or require an inpatient admission, whereas struck by/against injuries can often be treated in outpatient settings.

Total Lifetime Costs by Body Region, Severity, and Nature of Injury

Table 4.3 presents the total lifetime costs of injuries by body region. Upper-extremity and lower-extremity injuries each account for 17% ($68 billion) of the total costs of injuries. The vast majority, or 99%, of these costs are associated with hospitalized and nonhospitalized injuries. In contrast, 82% of the total costs of system-wide injuries are associated with fatal injuries. Figure 4.9 shows the distribution of total costs, by body region, between medical spending and lost productivity. For system-wide injuries, due to their high fatality rates, lost productivity accounts for 91% of the total costs. Even for severe nonfatal injuries that may require substantial rehabilitation, the costs of lost productivity substantially outweighs the costs of medical treatment: for example, medical spending accounts for only 31% of the total costs of SCIs.

Table 4.4 presents the total lifetime costs of injuries by nature of injury. Fractures, which represent 14% of the total incidence of injuries (Chapter 1), account for 24% ($99 billion) of the total costs of injuries: 3% ($5 billion) of the total costs of fatal injuries, 54% ($50 billion) of the total costs of hospitalized injuries, and 26% ($45 bil-

Table 4.3 Total Lifetime Costs of Injuries by Body Region, 2000 ($M)

	Fatal	Hospitalized	Nonhospitalized	Total
All	*$143,154*	*$92,453*	*$170,682*	*$406,289*
Traum brain inj	38,886	17,441	4,107	60,434
Other head/neck	4,377	6,561	24,068	35,006
Spinal cord inj	567	4,479	256	5,302
Vert column inj	448	3,940	19,745	24,133
Torso	20,570	8,451	13,911	42,932
Upper extremity	685	15,136	51,957	67,778
Lower extremity	1,268	30,043	37,159	68,470
Other/unspec	33,744	737	15,491	49,972
System-wide	42,610	5,665	3,988	52,263

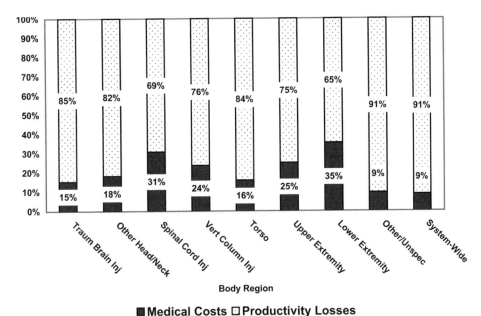

Figure 4.9 Distribution of Medical Costs and Productivity Losses, by Body Region

lion) of the total costs of nonhospitalized injuries. In comparison, injuries involving an open wound, which represent 18% of the incidence of injuries, account for 17% ($68 billion) of the total costs of injuries and 23% ($32 billion) of the total costs of fatal injuries. These relatively common injuries also account for 9% ($8 billion) and 16% ($27 billion) of the total costs of hospitalized and nonhospitalized injuries, respectively.

Table 4.4 Total Lifetime Costs of Injuries by Nature of Injury, 2000 ($M)

	Fatal	Hospitalized	Nonhospitalized	Total
All	*$143,154*	*$92,453*	*$170,682*	*$406,289*
Fracture	4,607	49,901	44,780	99,288
Dislocation	189	1,320	7,779	9,288
Sprain/strain	16	3,517	51,836	55,369
Internal organ	9,064	14,822	2,277	26,163
Open wound	32,276	7,891	27,498	67,665
Amputation	119	1,767	2,689	4,575
Blood vessel	1,743	442	25	2,210
Superfic/contusion	168	2,948	12,853	15,970
Crushing	768	264	1,192	2,224
Burn	1,084	1,254	3,772	6,110
Nerve	42	495	3,681	4,218
Unspecified	50,470	2,165	8,313	60,947
System-wide	42,610	5,665	3,988	52,263

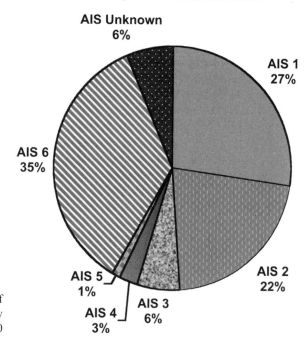

Figure 4.10 Distribution of Total Lifetime Costs by Severity, 2000

Figure 4.10 indicates that costs associated with AIS 1 and 2, or low severity, injuries ($111 billon and $87 billion, respectively) represent 85% of the injuries but only 49% of total injury costs. Both medical costs and productivity losses per episode are lower for these injuries. As a result, the share of costs associated with them is low compared to their high incidence. Conversely, AIS 6 injuries (fatal), which represent less than 1% of injuries, account for 35% of the total costs. The high costs of fatal injuries is largely explained by their relatively high productivity losses.

Patterns of Total Lifetime Costs by Mechanism

The following section describes the total costs of injuries separately for 8 major mechanisms, stratified by age and sex.

Motor Vehicle/Other Road User

Figure 4.11 shows the total lifetime costs of motor vehicle injuries by age and sex. Motor vehicle injuries, which represent only 10% of the incidence of injuries, account for 22% of the total costs of injuries, or $89 billion. Overall, males account for $64 billion, or 72% of the total costs of motor-vehicle injuries; females account for $25 billion, or 28% of the total costs of motor-vehicle injuries. For both males and females, those aged 25 to 44 years account for the highest percentage of total costs; persons 25 to 44, who represent only 30% of the U.S. population, account for 43% ($28 billion) of the total costs of motor-vehicle injuries among males and 40%

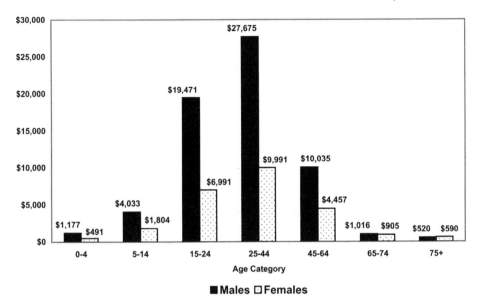

Figure 4.11 Total Lifetime Costs of Motor Vehicle Injuries by Age and Sex, 2000 ($M)

($10 billion) of the total costs among females. Similarly, persons aged 15 to 24, who represent only 14% of the U.S. population, account for 30% ($19 billion) of the total costs of motor-vehicle injuries among males and 28% ($7 billion) of the total costs of motor-vehicle injuries among females.

Figure 4.12 shows the total lifetime costs of fatal, hospitalized, and nonhospitalized motor-vehicle injuries by age and sex. Fatal motor-vehicle injuries total $47 billion, or 33% of the total costs of fatal injuries; hospitalized motor-vehicle injuries total $24 billion, or 26% of the total costs of hospitalized injuries; and nonhospitalized motor-vehicle injuries total $19 billion, or 11% of the total costs of nonhospitalized injuries (Table 4.2). Although the costs of fatal and hospitalized motor vehicle injuries is largely borne by males (males account for more than 70% of the total costs of fatal and hospitalized injuries), the costs of nonhospitalized injuries, especially for persons aged 15 to 64 years, is more evenly distributed between males and females: for example, males and females aged 15 to 24 years account for 52% ($1.9 billion) and 48% ($1.8 billion) of the total costs of nonhospitalized injuries for that age group, respectively. This result is largely driven by the fact that nonhospitalized injuries are unlikely to be associated with prolonged productivity losses, which disproportionately increase productivity costs for males.

Falls

Figure 4.13 shows the total lifetime costs of fall injuries by age and sex. Fall injuries, which represent 23% of the incidence of injuries, account for 20% of the total costs of injuries, or $81 billion (Table 4.2). For both males ($44 billion) and females ($37 billion), the total costs of fall injuries are substantial. In fact, among females, fall injuries account for a higher percentage of total costs (30%) than does any other

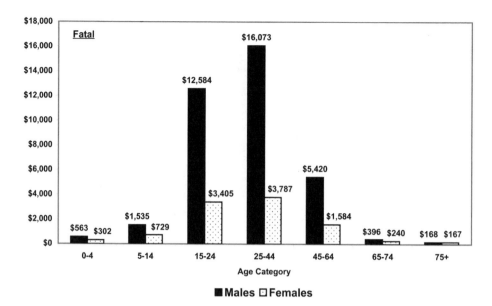

Figure 4.12a Total Lifetime Costs of Fatal Motor-Vehicle Injuries by Age and Sex, 2000 ($M)

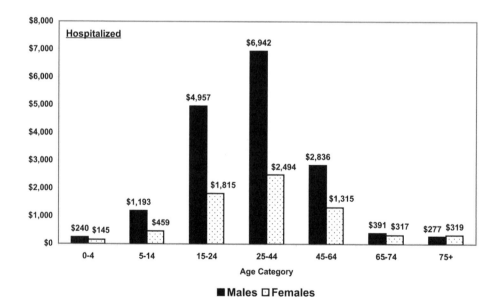

Figure 4.12b Total Lifetime Costs of Hospitalized Motor-Vehicle Injuries by Age and Sex, 2000 ($M)

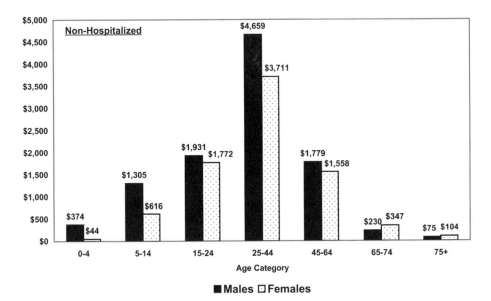

Figure 4.12c Total Lifetime Costs of Nonhospitalized Motor-Vehicle Injuries by Age and Sex, 2000 ($M)

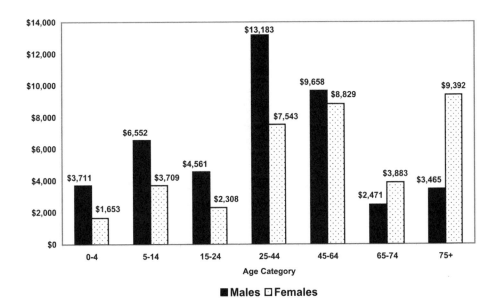

Figure 4.13 Total Lifetime Costs of Fall Injuries by Age and Sex, 2000 ($M)

mechanism; among males, only motor-vehicle injuries account for a higher percentage of total costs. For males, the total costs of fall injuries are highest among persons aged 25 to 45 years; males in this age group, who represent 30% of the U.S. male population, account for 30% ($13 billion) of the total costs of fall injuries among males. For females, the total costs of fall injuries are highest among persons age 75 years and greater; females in this age group, who represent 7% of the U.S. female population, account for 25% ($9 billion) of the total costs of fall injuries among females. In fact, fall injuries account for nearly 76% of the total costs of injuries for females age 75 years and greater.

Figure 4.14 shows the total costs of fatal, hospitalized, and nonhospitalized fall injuries by age and sex. Fatal fall injuries total $5 billion, or 3% of the total costs of fatal injuries; hospitalized fall injuries total $34 billion, or 36% of the total costs of hospitalized injuries; and nonhospitalized fall injuries total $42 billion, or 25% of the total costs of nonhospitalized injuries. Although males account for nearly 80% of the total costs of fatal fall injuries, the total costs of hospitalized and nonhospitalized fall injuries are distributed almost equally between males and females; males account for 52% and 53% of the total costs of hospitalized and nonhospitalized fall injuries, respectively. The total costs of fall injuries among males are highest for persons aged 25 to 44 years, and the total costs of fall injuries among females are highest for those age 75 years and greater.

Struck by/against

Figure 4.15 shows the total costs of struck by/against injuries by age and sex. Struck by/against injuries, which represent 21% of the incidence of injuries, account for

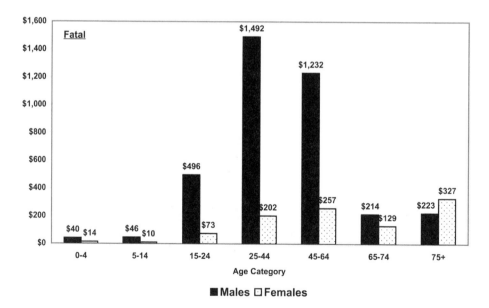

Figure 4.14a Total Lifetime Costs of Fatal Fall Injuries by Age and Sex, 2000 ($M)

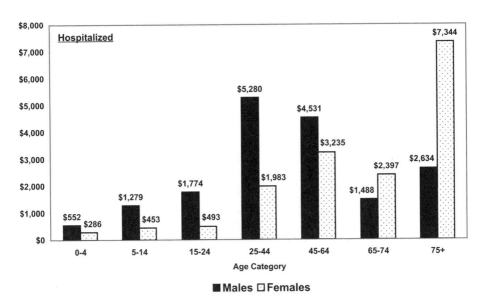

Figure 4.14b Total Lifetime Costs of Hospitalized Fall Injuries by Age and Sex, 2000 ($M)

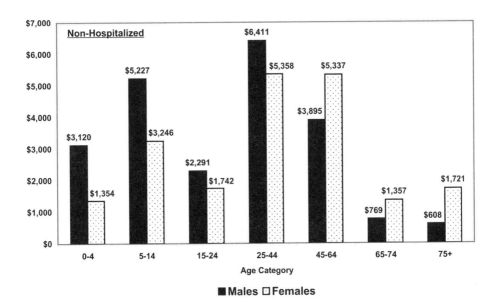

Figure 4.14c Total Lifetime Costs of Nonhospitalized Fall Injuries by Age and Sex, 2000 ($M)

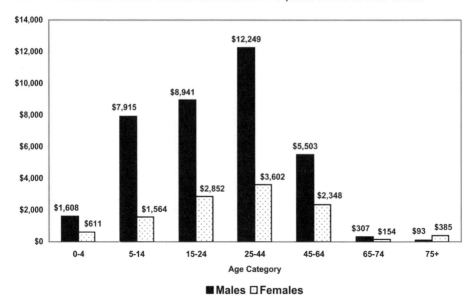

Figure 4.15 Total Lifetime Costs of Struck by/against Injuries by Age and Sex, 2000 ($M)

only 12% of the total costs of injuries, or $48 billion. Overall, males account for $37 billion, or 76% of the total costs of struck by/against injuries; females account for $12 billion, or 24%. For all ages under 75 years, males had higher total costs associated with struck by/against injuries compared to females, with the greatest differential evident in persons aged 5 to 14, where the total struck by/against injury-related costs for males was more than 5 times higher than the total costs for females.

Figure 4.16 shows the total costs of fatal, hospitalized, and nonhospitalized struck by/against injuries by age and sex. Fatal struck by/against injuries total $1 billion, or 1% of the total costs of fatal injuries; hospitalized struck by/against injuries total $6 billion, or 7% of the total costs of hospitalized injuries; and non-hospitalized struck by/against injuries total $40 billion, or 24% of the total costs of nonhospitalized injuries. Males account for more than 85% of the total costs of both fatal and hospitalized struck by/against injuries; however, even among males, struck by/against injuries account for only a small fraction of the total costs of fatal and hospitalized injuries. The total costs that result from nonhospitalized struck by/against injuries, on the other hand, are substantial. In fact, for males aged 5 to 44 years, struck by/against nonhospitalized injuries account for 49% ($23.7 billion) of the total costs for all struck by/against injuries.

Cut/Pierce

Figure 4.17 shows the total costs of cut/pierce injuries by age and sex. Cut/pierce injuries, which represent 8% of the incidence of injuries, account for only 4% of the total costs of injuries, or $16 billion. Overall, males account for $12 billion, or 75% of the total costs of cut/pierce injuries; females account for $4 billion, or 25% of the

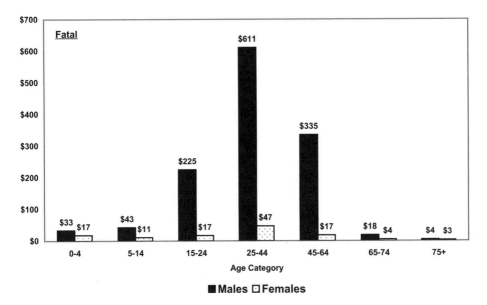

Figure 4.16a Total Lifetime Costs of Fatal Struck by/against Injuries by Age and Sex, 2000 ($M)

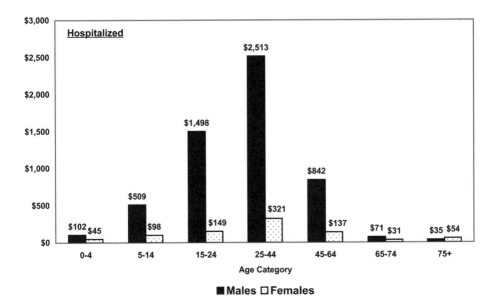

Figure 4.16b Total Lifetime Costs of Hospitalized Struck by/against Injuries by Age and Sex, 2000 ($M)

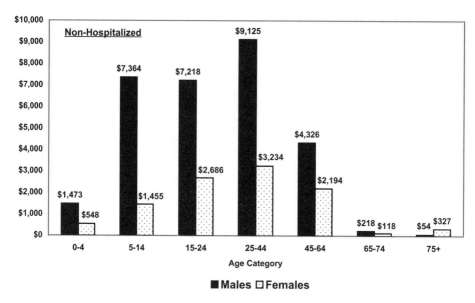

Figure 4.16c Total Lifetime Costs of Nonhospitalized Struck by/against Injuries by Age and Sex, 2000 ($M)

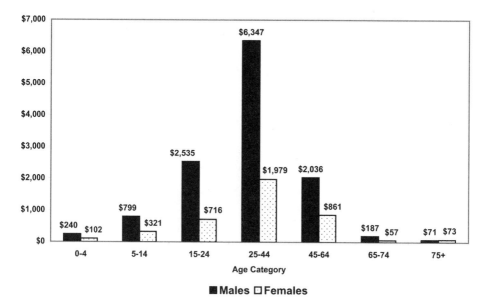

Figure 4.17 Total Lifetime Costs of Cut/Pierce Injuries by Age and Sex, 2000 ($M)

146

total costs of cut/pierce injuries. For both males and females, persons aged 25 to 44 years, who represent 30% of the U.S. population, account for roughly half of the total costs of cut/pierce injuries: males aged 25 to 44 years account for 52% ($6 billion), and females aged 25 to 44 years account for 48% ($2 billion).

Figure 4.18 shows the total costs of fatal, hospitalized, and nonhospitalized cut/pierce injuries by age and sex. Fatal cut/pierce injuries total $3 billion, or 2% of the total costs of fatal injuries; hospitalized cut/pierce injuries total $4 billion, or 5% of the total costs of hospitalized injuries; and nonhospitalized cut/pierce injuries total $9 billion, or 6% of the total costs of nonhospitalized injuries. In general, the total costs of cut/pierce injuries among males, regardless of injury category, is higher than that among females; however, even for males, cut/pierce injuries account for only a small fraction of the total costs of fatal, hospitalized, and nonhospitalized injuries.

Fire/Burn

Figure 4.19 shows the total costs of fire/burn injuries by age and sex. Fire/burn injuries, which represent 1% of the incidence of injuries, account for 2% of the total costs of injuries, or $7.5 billion. Overall, males account for $5 billion, or 64% of the total costs of fire/burn injuries; females account for $3 billion, or 36% of the total costs of fire/burn injuries.

Figure 4.20 shows the total costs of fatal, hospitalized, and nonhospitalized fire/burn injuries by age and sex. Fatal fire/burn injuries total $3 billion, or 2% of the total costs of fatal injuries; hospitalized fire/burn injuries total $1 billion, or 1% of

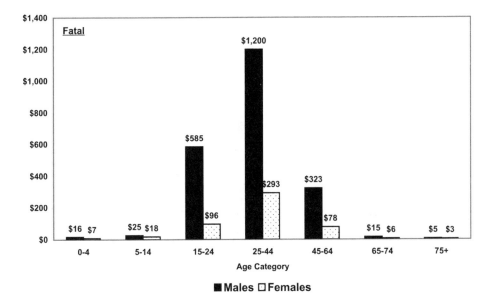

Figure 4.18a Total Lifetime Costs of Fatal Cut/Pierce Injuries by Age and Sex, 2000 ($M)

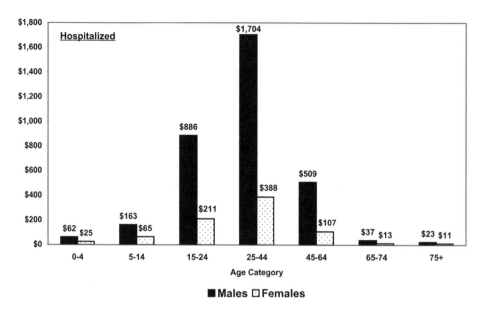

Figure 4.18b Total Lifetime Costs of Hospitalized Cut/Pierce Injuries by Age and Sex, 2000 ($M)

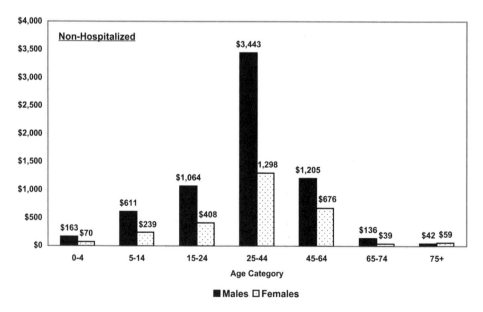

Figure 4.18c Total Lifetime Costs of Nonhospitalized Cut/Pierce Injuries by Age and Sex, 2000 ($M)

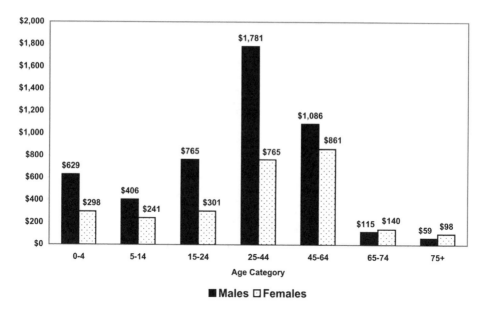

Figure 4.19 Total Lifetime Costs of Fire/Burn Injuries by Age and Sex, 2000 ($M)

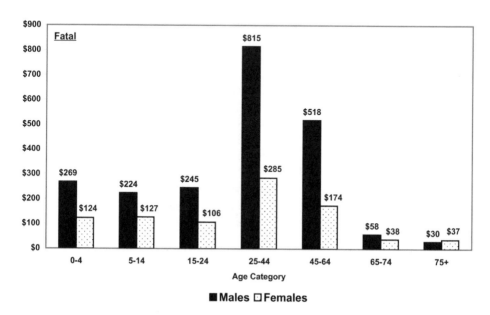

Figure 4.20a Total Lifetime Costs of Fatal Fire/Burn Injuries by Age and Sex, 2000 ($M)

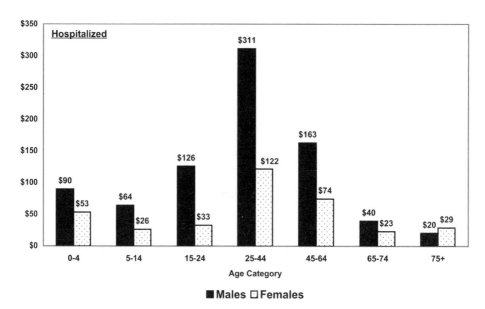

Figure 4.20b Total Lifetime Costs of Hospitalized Fire/Burn Injuries by Age and Sex, 2000 ($M)

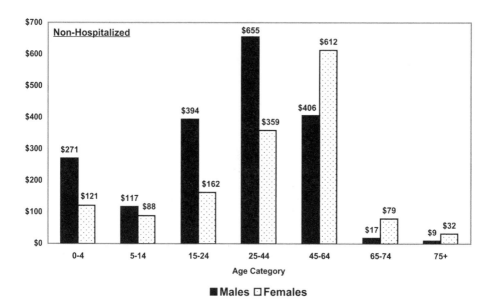

Figure 4.20c Total Lifetime Costs of Nonhospitalized Fire/Burn Injuries by Age and Sex, 2000 ($M)

the total costs of hospitalized injuries; and nonhospitalized fire/burn injuries total $3 billion, or 2% of the total costs of nonhospitalized injuries. For fatal and hospitalized fires/burns, males had higher lifetime costs than females for all age categories except those aged 75 years and older. For nonhospitalized fires/burns, males had higher lifetime costs than females up through age 44, after which the trend is reversed.

Poisonings

Figure 4.21 shows the total costs of poisoning injuries by age and sex. Poisoning injuries, which represent 2.5% of the incidence of injuries, account for 6% of the total costs of injuries, or $26 billion. Overall, males account for $19 billion, or 75% of the total costs of poisoning injuries; females account for almost $7 billion, or 25% of the total costs of poisoning injuries. For males and females, those aged 25 to 44 years, who represent 30% of the U.S. population, account for 62% and 55% of the gender-specific total costs of poisoning injuries, respectively.

Figure 4.22 shows the total costs of fatal, hospitalized, and nonhospitalized poisoning injuries by age and sex. Although males account for a higher percentage of the total costs of fatal (78%) and nonhospitalized (54%) poisoning injuries than females, females account for a higher percentage (53%) of the total costs of hospitalized poisoning injuries. Fatal poisoning injuries total $23 billion, or 16% of the total costs of fatal injuries; hospitalized poisoning injuries total $2 billion, or 2% of the total costs of hospitalized injuries; and nonhospitalized poisoning injuries total $1 billion, or 1% of the total costs of nonhospitalized injuries.

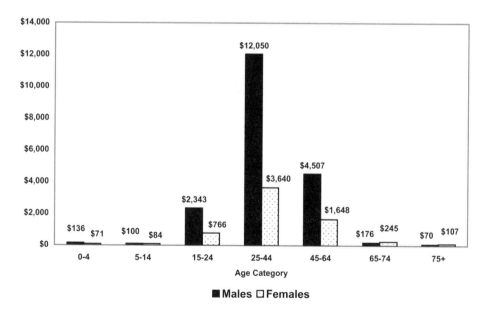

Figure 4.21 Total Lifetime Costs of Poisoning Injuries by Age and Sex, 2000 ($M)

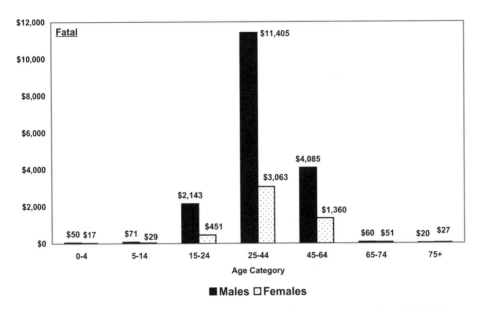

Figure 4.22a Total Lifetime Costs of Fatal Poisoning Injuries by Age and Sex, 2000 ($M)

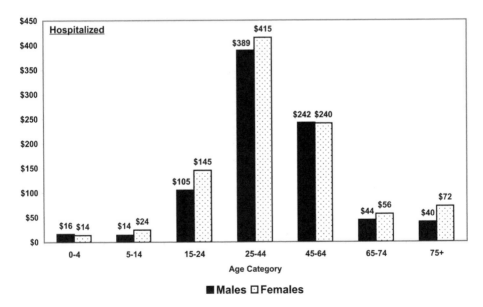

Figure 4.22b Total Lifetime Costs of Hospitalized Poisoning Injuries by Age and Sex, 2000 ($M)

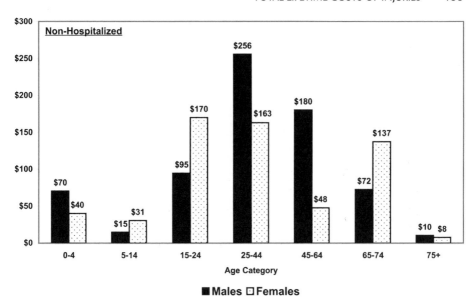

Figure 4.22c Total Lifetime Costs of Nonhospitalized Poisoning Injuries by Age and Sex, 2000 ($M)

Drowning/Submersion

Figure 4.23 shows the total costs of drowning injuries by age and sex. Fatal and nonfatal drownings account for less than 1% of both injury incidence and total costs ($5 billion). Overall, males account for $4 billion, or 84% of the total costs of drowning injuries; females account for less than $1 billion, or 16% of the total costs of these injuries.

Figure 4.24 shows the total costs of fatal and hospitalized drowning/submersion injuries by age and sex (note: nonfatal, nonhospitalized drowning/submersion injuries are extremely rare). Fatal drowning/submersion injuries total $5 billion, or 3% of the total costs of fatal injuries; and hospitalized drowning/submersion injuries total less than $1 billion, or less than 1% of the total costs of hospitalized injuries. Females aged 0 to 4 years, who represent 7% of the U.S. female population, account for 27% and 36% of the total costs of fatal and hospitalized drowning injuries, among females respectively; females aged 5 to 14 years, who represent 14% of the U.S. female population, account for 26% of hospitalized drowning injuries among females. Similarly, males aged 0 to 4 years, who account for 8% of the U.S. male population, account for 31% of hospitalized drowning injuries among males.

Firearm/Gunshot

Figure 4.25 shows the total costs of firearm/gunshot injuries by age and sex. Firearm/gunshot injuries, which represent less than 1% of incidence of injuries, account for 9% of the total costs of injuries, or $36 billion. Overall, males account for $33 billion, or 90% of the total costs of firearm/gunshot injuries; females account for

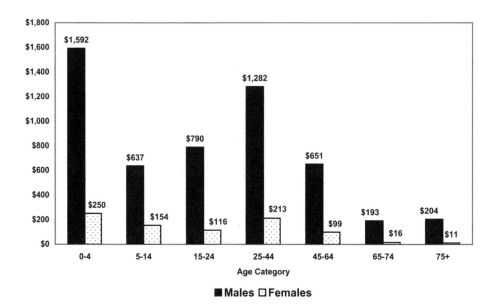

Figure 4.23 Total Lifetime Costs of Drowning/Submersion Injuries by Age and Sex, 2000 ($M)

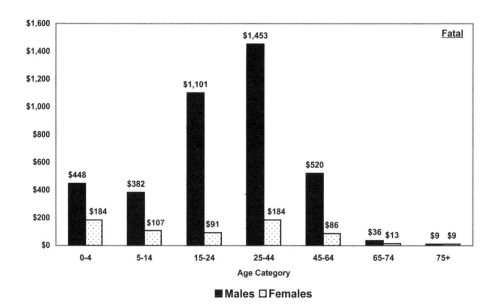

Figure 4.24a Total Lifetime Costs of Fatal Drowning/Submersion Injuries by Age and Sex, 2000 ($M)

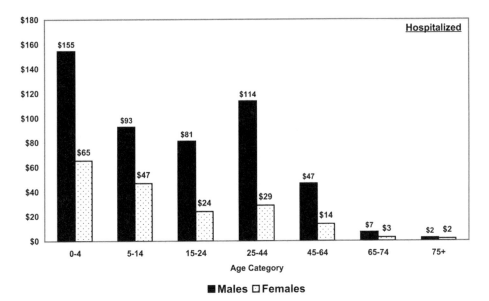

Figure 4.24b Total Lifetime Costs of Hospitalized Drowning/Submersion Injuries by Age and Sex, 2000 ($M)

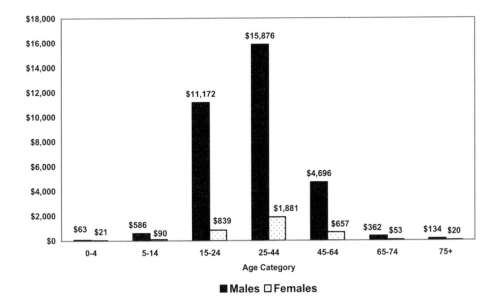

Figure 4.25 Total Lifetime Costs of Firearm/Gunshot Injuries by Age and Sex, 2000 ($M)

155

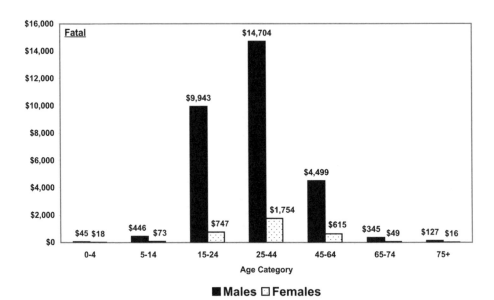

Figure 4.26a Total Lifetime Costs of Fatal Firearm/Gunshot Injuries by Age and Sex, 2000 ($M)

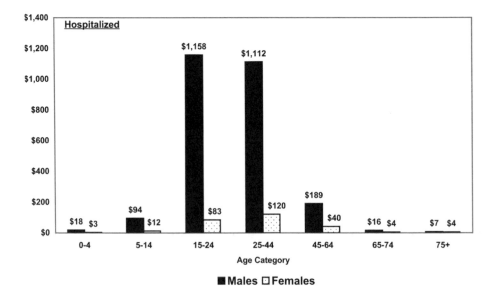

Figure 4.26b Total Lifetime Costs of Hospitalized Firearm/Gunshot Injuries by Age and Sex, 2000 ($M)

$3.6 billion, or 10% of the total costs of firearm/gunshot injuries. More than 80% of the combined total costs for males and females results from firearm/gunshot injuries among persons aged 15 to 44 years.

Figure 4.26 shows the total costs of fatal and hospitalized firearm/gunshot injuries by age and sex (note: nonfatal, nonhospitalized firearm/gunshot injuries are extremely rare). Fatal firearm/gunshot injuries total $33 billion, or 23% of the total costs of fatal injuries; hospitalized firearm/gunshot injuries total $3 billion, or 3% of the total costs of hospitalized injuries. Firearm/gunshot injuries account for a substantial portion of the total costs of fatal injuries among males for all age groups with the exception of those aged 0 to 4. Estimates range from 13% for those aged 5 to 14 years to 32% for those aged 15 to 24 years.

Summary

Injuries represent a substantial burden to society. As this chapter demonstrates, burden can be considered along several dimensions: including incidence, medical costs, productivity losses, or total costs. The relative burden of specific classes of injuries (e.g., by mechanism, age, gender) varies depending upon the perspective chosen. As we discuss in the following chapter, differing perspectives about the relative burden of injuries across classes or when compared to other medical conditions may impact resource allocation decisions and injury prevention efforts.

Appendix 4.1 Unit (Total) Cost of Injuries, by Age, Sex, and Treatment Location

Age and Sex	Fatal Injuries	Hospitalized	ED Treated	Outpatient	Doctor's Office	Total
All	*$960,283*	*$49,444*	*$3,548*	*$3,520*	*$3,468*	*$8,074*
0–4	1,029,276	55,069	2,666	2,442	3,441	4,667
5–14	1,264,506	65,166	3,318	3,006	2,629	4,329
15–24	1,554,953	75,315	3,202	2,824	2,763	9,021
25–44	1,409,357	71,807	4,269	4,376	4,090	10,468
45–64	803,845	54,777	4,094	4,017	4,452	9,101
65–74	205,559	31,249	2,424	2,140	2,399	5,604
75+	64,784	21,700	1,658	1,356	1,880	5,768
Male	*$1,129,484*	*$67,428*	*$4,017*	*$3,934*	*$4,259*	*$10,658*
0–4	1,193,513	63,304	3,023	3,004	4,191	5,373
5–14	1,433,397	75,113	3,749	3,202	3,327	5,237
15–24	1,675,474	91,033	3,515	3,105	3,318	11,946
25–44	1,541,408	87,056	4,834	4,837	4,908	14,152
45–64	890,968	66,029	4,639	4,642	5,789	12,738
65–74	212,358	35,057	2,499	2,353	2,647	6,231
75+	60,468	23,737	1,667	1,204	1,640	5,681
Female	*$571,130*	*$32,691*	*$2,956*	*$3,062*	*$2,699*	*$5,160*
0–4	799,701	43,791	2,180	1,742	—	3,578
5–14	963,292	47,488	2,661	2,722	1,873	3,118
15–24	1,114,246	46,123	2,713	2,393	2,177	4,953
25–44	977,834	46,130	3,512	3,845	3,236	5,967
45–64	568,274	41,387	3,550	3,509	3,363	5,778
65–74	192,778	28,811	2,371	1,956	2,180	5,105
75+	69,060	20,971	1,654	1,399	1,997	5,808

Appendix 4.2 Unit (Total) Cost of Injuries, by Body Region, Sex, and Treatment Location

Body Region	Fatal Injuries	Hospitalized	ED Treated	Outpatient	Doctor's Office	Total
All	*$960,283*	*$49,444*	*$3,548*	*$3,520*	*$3,468*	*$8,074*
Traum brain inj	968,557	112,095	3,816	3,188	2,345	44,986
Other head/neck	951,189	45,534	3,822	3,064	3,575	5,347
Spinal cord inj	746,207	434,218	16,008	—	—	195,918
Vert column inj	584,483	45,700	4,342	4,193	4,082	5,051
Torso	889,550	34,542	3,545	3,642	3,485	10,274
Upper extremity	774,364	54,979	4,057	4,066	3,793	5,065
Lower extremity	172,713	45,783	3,064	3,824	3,961	6,053
Other/unspec	1,042,610	40,147	2,884	2,631	2,412	8,522
System-wide	1,090,174	20,296	1,719	1,358	1,183	17,737

Appendix 4.3 Unit (Total) Cost of Injuries, by Nature, Sex, and Treatment Location

Nature of Injury	Fatal Injuries	Hospitalized	ED Treated	Outpatient	Doctor's Office	Total
Total	*$960,283*	*$49,444*	*$3,548*	*$3,520*	*$3,468*	*$8,074*
Fracture	378,906	54,210	7,528	7,234	7,096	14,121
Dislocation	884,502	59,202	5,479	6,443	5,764	6,686
Sprain/strain	1,056,253	43,948	3,644	3,448	3,223	3,626
Internal organ	739,994	79,214	5,740	4,609	5,456	43,642
Open wound	1,154,389	50,829	3,290	2,936	2,502	7,576
Amputation	1,120,360	231,308	42,110	38,461	34,247	62,100
Blood vessel	834,242	74,825	5,461	1,478	952	97,216
Superfic/contusion	592,493	21,571	1,425	1,358	885	1,516
Crushing	1,052,373	85,677	6,329	5,255	6,996	11,896
Burn	1,039,995	47,124	5,266	3,893	4,339	7,687
Nerve	886,443	103,534	79,058	8,589	33,099	40,177
Unspecified	950,517	53,048	3,498	3,315	2,821	23,246
System-wide	1,090,174	20,296	1,719	1,358	1,183	17,737

Chapter 5

The Burden of Injuries

Trends and Implications

Injuries in the United States have an enormous impact on society. The results presented in Chapter 4 reveal that the total costs for the roughly 50 million injuries that occurred in 2000 exceed $400 billion. This burden is shared by individuals, families, employers, and communities. For example, medical costs of injury are paid by individuals, private insurers, and, to a large extent, taxpayers who indirectly fund government health insurance programs. Likewise, work loss costs, while imposing the greatest burden on victims and their families, also burden insurance and public welfare programs. The financial impact of short-term work loss is often absorbed by employers, and long-term work loss due to permanent injury-associated disability is split into unknown proportions between victims, private and public insurers, and public welfare programs. An understanding of how the incidence and costs of injuries are distributed among certain subpopulations can be used to design targeted prevention strategies to minimize the burden of injuries on society.

Burden Comparisons

Table 5.1 shows incidence counts, rates (per 100,000), and lifetime costs of fatal and nonfatal injuries by sex and age category. Persons aged 25 to 44 years have the highest number of injury-attributable fatalities, while persons aged 75 years and older have the highest rate of injury-attributable fatalities. Among males, those aged 25 to

Table 5.1 Incidence Counts and Rates (per 100,000) and Total Lifetime Costs of Injuries by Age Category and Sex, 2000

| | Fatal | | Total | | Costs ($M) | | |
| | | | | | Medical Costs | Productivity Losses | Total Costs |
	Incidence	Rate	Incidence	Rate			
Total	*149,075*	*54*	*50,127,098*	*18,135*	*$80,248*	*$326,042*	*$406,289*
0–4	3,532	18	3,426,571	17,403	3,729	12,264	15,992
5–14	3,741	9	7,945,792	19,249	8,170	26,400	34,569
15–24	23,698	63	8,818,414	23,604	12,895	66,940	79,835
25–44	48,487	59	15,553,007	18,818	22,704	141,188	163,892
45–64	31,935	53	8,814,553	14,750	14,278	66,311	80,589
65–74	10,595	60	2,379,274	13,488	5,865	7,541	13,406
75+	27,087	179	3,189,486	21,067	12,608	5,399	18,007
Male	*103,900*	*77*	*26,565,230*	*19,736*	*$44,445*	*$238,688*	*$283,133*
0–4	2,059	20	2,079,034	20,244	2,438	8,733	11,170
5–14	2,397	11	4,541,429	21,688	4,973	18,810	23,783
15–24	18,609	98	5,129,575	27,026	8,346	52,930	61,276
25–44	37,126	92	8,553,856	21,215	14,033	107,019	121,052
45–64	23,313	81	4,208,735	14,558	7,999	45,612	53,611
65–74	6,916	87	1,055,713	13,215	2,704	3,873	6,578
75+	13,480	228	996,889	16,827	3,952	1,712	5,663
Female	*45,175*	*32*	*23,561,868*	*16,616*	*$35,803*	*$87,353*	*$123,156*
0–4	1,473	16	1,347,538	14,311	1,291	3,531	4,822
5–14	1,344	7	3,404,363	16,737	3,197	7,589	10,786
15–24	5,089	28	3,688,839	20,059	4,549	14,010	18,559
25–44	11,361	27	6,999,151	16,535	8,671	34,169	42,840
45–64	8,622	28	4,605,818	14,930	6,279	20,699	26,978
65–74	3,679	38	1,323,561	13,711	3,160	3,668	6,828
75+	13,607	148	2,192,597	23,783	8,656	3,687	12,343

44 years have the highest number of injury-attributable fatalities, while among females, those aged 75 years and older have the highest number of injury-attributable fatalities. For both fatal and nonfatal injuries, males and females aged 25 to 44 years have the highest number of injuries. However, males aged 15 to 24 and females aged 75 years and older have the highest rate of injuries.

Similar to incidence, persons aged 25 to 44 years incur the greatest burden of lifetime medical costs ($22.7 billion), a burden 50% greater than that of any other age category. For males, the medical cost burden for persons aged 25 to 44 years ($14 billion) is more than 60% higher than that of any other age category. For females, the medical cost burden among persons aged 25 to 44 years or 75 years and older (at $8.7 billion each) is higher than that of any other age category. Defining burden by losses in productivity suggests a similar pattern for persons of both sexes, that is, persons aged 25 to 44 years incur the greatest productivity loss burden ($141 billion).

Exploring burden estimates by mechanism is also important for targeting prevention policies and programs. Table 5.2 highlights incidence counts, rates (per 100,000), and lifetime costs of injuries by sex and mechanism.

Motor-vehicle/other road-user injuries resulted in the highest number and rate of injury fatalities, followed by firearm/gunshot, and poisoning. The same ordering holds

Table 5.2 Incidence Counts and Rates (per 100,000) and Total Lifetime Costs of Injuries by Mechanism and Sex, 2000

	Fatal		Total		Costs ($M)		
					Medical Costs	Productivity Losses	Total Costs
	Incidence	Rate	Incidence	Rate			
Total	*149,075*	*54*	*50,127,098*	*18,135*	*$80,248*	*$326,042*	*$406,289*
MV/other road user	43,802	16	5,010,439	1,813	14,026	75,130	89,156
Falls	14,052	5	11,566,742	4,185	26,892	54,028	80,920
Struck by/against	1,301	0	10,674,180	3,862	11,028	37,104	48,132
Cut/pierce	2,293	1	4,124,085	1,492	3,662	12,664	16,326
Fire/burn	3,922	1	774,376	280	1,345	6,202	7,546
Poisoning	20,261	7	1,267,465	459	2,236	23,707	25,944
Drowning/submersion	4,168	2	10,083	4	95	5,215	5,310
Firearm/gunshot	28,722	10	131,013	47	1,225	35,226	36,451
Other/unclassified*	30,554	11	16,568,716	5,994	19,738	76,767	96,505
Male	*103,900*	*77*	*26,565,232*	*19,736*	*$44,445*	*$238,688*	*$283,133*
MV/other road user	29,686	22	2,551,330	1,895	8,713	55,214	63,927
Falls	7,647	6	5,201,676	3,865	11,778	31,824	43,602
Struck by/against	1,109	1	6,660,301	4,948	7,493	29,123	36,617
Cut/pierce	1,678	1	2,602,084	1,933	2,442	9,775	12,217
Fire/Burn	2,333	2	371,988	276	764	4,078	4,842
Poisoning	13,721	10	588,900	438	1,063	18,319	19,382
Drowning/submersion	3,198	2	7,016	5	61	4,389	4,450
Firearm/gunshot	24,638	18	117,029	87	1,081	31,809	32,890
Other/unclassified*	19,890	15	8,464,908	6,289	11,050	54,157	65,207
Female	*45,175*	*32*	*23,561,868*	*16,616*	*$35,803*	*$87,353*	*$123,156*
MV/other road user	14,116	10	2,459,105	1,734	5,313	19,916	25,229
Falls	6,405	5	6,365,066	4,489	15,114	22,204	37,318
Struck by/against	192	0	4,013,880	2,831	3,535	7,981	11,516
Cut/pierce	615	0	1,522,001	1,073	1,221	2,889	4,109
Fire/burn	1,589	1	402,389	284	581	2,124	2,704
Poisoning	6,540	5	678,565	479	1,173	5,388	6,562
Drowning/submersion	970	1	3,067	2	34	825	859
Firearm/gunshot	4,084	3	13,984	10	144	3,417	3,561
Other/unclassified*	10,664	8	8,103,807	5,715	8,688	22,610	31,298

*Injuries categorized as "other" resulted from varied mechanisms: for fatal injuries, these other mechanisms primarily resulted from inhalation/suffocation (8%) and unspecified (8%); for hospitalized injuries, these other mechanisms primarily resulted from unspecified mechanisms (5%), and overexertion (2%), and other transport (2%); for less severe nonhospitalized injuries, these other mechanisms primarily resulted from overexertion (11%), bite/sting (7%), and other transport (2%).

for males, while motor-vehicle/other road-user injuries, poisonings, and falls resulted in the highest number and rate of injury fatalities for females. Falls and struck by/against injuries resulted in the highest combined incidence and rate for all fatal and nonfatal injuries. For males, struck by/against injuries resulted in the highest number of total injuries; for females, falls resulted in the highest number of total injuries.

When the burden of injuries is defined by lifetime medical costs, falls represent the greatest burden, $27 billion, which is more than 90% greater than the lifetime medical costs of the next highest mechanism (motor vehicle/other road user, $14 billion). The same pattern for medical cost burden holds for males and females. In contrast, motor-vehicle/other road-user injuries represent the most substantial burden related to productivity losses ($75 billion) and total lifetime costs ($89 billion), followed by falls ($54 billion in productivity losses, and $81 billion in total costs). While these patterns hold for males, for females, falls result in greater productivity losses ($22 billion in productivity losses, and $37 billion in total costs) than motor-vehicle/other road-user injuries ($20 billion in productivity losses, and $25 billion in total costs).

Limited resources dedicated to injury prevention force policy makers to make difficult decisions concerning the appropriate level of resources to dedicate towards preventing one type of injury or another. Understanding the relative burden that injuries impose on society can help policy makers develop targeted prevention strategies to ameliorate that burden. Although burden estimates do not provide information about how effective or cost-effective prevention strategies might be, they help policy makers identify and target areas for improvement. Whether policy makers focus on one, or a combination of these burden measures, may ultimately determine how scarce resources are allocated.

Figure 5.1 compares the relative burden of injury—defined as incidence, medical costs, productivity losses, or total costs—by mechanism. The figure reveals, for example, that motor-vehicle injuries account for 10% of the incidence of injuries but 22% of the total costs. If one were to allocate injury prevention dollars based on incidence alone, the amount allocated towards reducing motor-vehicle injuries might be less than had both incidence and total costs been considered together. In contrast, struck by/against injuries, which account for 22% of the incidence of injuries, only account for 12% of the total costs, suggesting that these injuries, while more numerous, are less severe in nature.

The distribution of burden for falls shows that incidence and medical costs are disproportionately high relative to total costs, when compared to all other mechanisms. This results because falls are more likely to occur in age groups that do not experience heavy productivity losses (i.e., the young and the old) (see Table 5.3).

Comparison to 1989 Report

Allocating resources toward injury prevention overall, or for select mechanisms, may depend largely on trends in injury incidence over time. Authors of the 1989 report to Congress [Rice et al. 1989] concluded that the rate of medically-treated injuries in 1985 was 21,330 per 100,000. We estimate that in 2000, this rate was 18,135 per 100,000, a reduction of about 15%.

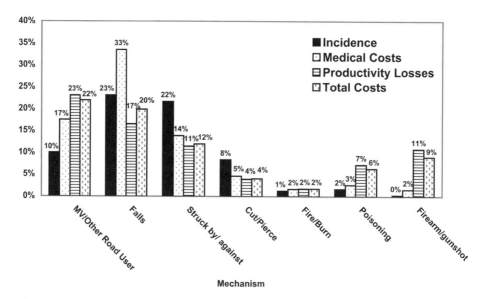

Figure 5.1 Distribution of Injury Incidence, Medical Costs, Productivity Losses, and Total Costs by Mechanism, 2000

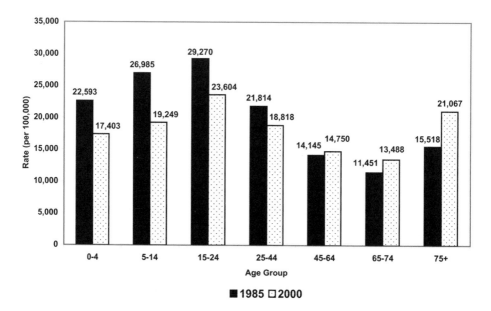

Figure 5.2 The Incidence Rate of Injuries (per 100,000) by Age Category, 1985 vs. 2000

Figure 5.2 compares the incidence rates (per 100,000) of all injuries by age category, estimated for 1985 and 2000. For those aged 0 to 44, the incidence rate of injuries declined by more than 20% from 1985 to 2000. In contrast, the incidence rate of injuries among those older than age 45 increased. The increase was highest, nearly 20%, for those persons aged 75 years and older.

Figures 5.3, 5.4, and 5.5 show the incidence rates (per 100,000) of fatal, hospitalized, and nonhospitalized injuries, respectively, by age group for 1985 and 2000. The rate of fatal injuries (Figure 5.3) decreased from 1985 to 2000 for every age category except for persons aged 75 years and older (with an increase of 11%). The rate of hospitalized injuries (Figure 5.4) decreased from 1985 to 2000 for all age categories except for 65 to 74 years (with an increase of 1%) and 75 years and greater (with an increase of 28%). The rate of nonhospitalized injuries (Figure 5.5) decreased by 12% to 28% from 1985 to 2000 for all age categories younger than age 45 and increased by 7% to 38% for all age categories 45 years and older.

Figure 5.6 compares the rate of injuries per 100,000 persons in 1985 and 2000 for five mechanism categories created using identical definitions. The figure shows a decline in the rate of injuries since 1985 for all five mechanisms. Firearm/gunshot and fire/burn injuries each decreased by more than 50%. Poisonings decreased by almost 30%. Motor-vehicle and fall injuries decreased by 5% and 10%, respectively.

Figures 5.7, 5.8, and 5.9 show the incidence rates (per 100,000) of fatal, hospitalized, and nonhospitalized injuries, respectively, by mechanism for 1985 and 2000. For rates of fatal injuries (Figure 5.7), poisoning was the only mechanism to show an increase (40%) from 1985 to 2000. The growth in poisoning deaths resulted in part from reclassification of unintentional drug overdoses as poisoning deaths in ICD-10. For hospitalized injuries (Figure 5.8), rates have declined for all mechanisms since 1985, with the biggest declines evident for firearms (60%), fire/burns (60%),

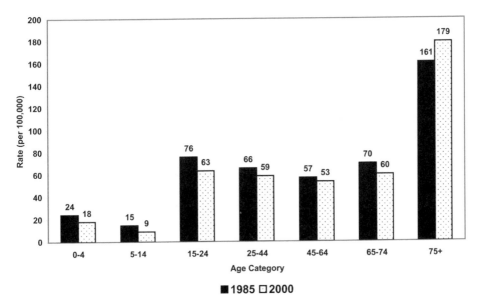

Figure 5.3 The Incidence Rate of Fatal Injuries (per 100,000) by Age Category, 1985 vs. 2000

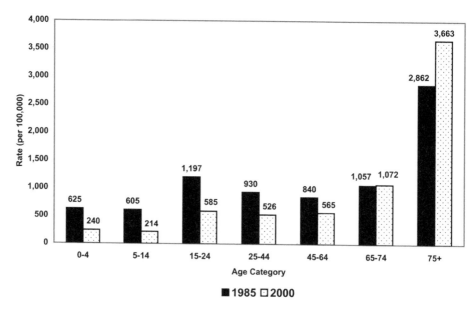

Figure 5.4 The Incidence Rate of Hospitalized Injuries (per 100,000) by Age Category, 1985 vs. 2000

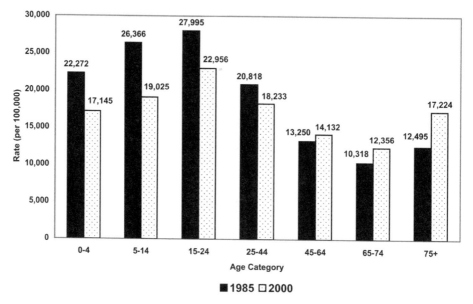

Figure 5.5 The Incidence Rate of Nonhospitalized Injuries (per 100,000) by Age Category, 1985 vs. 2000

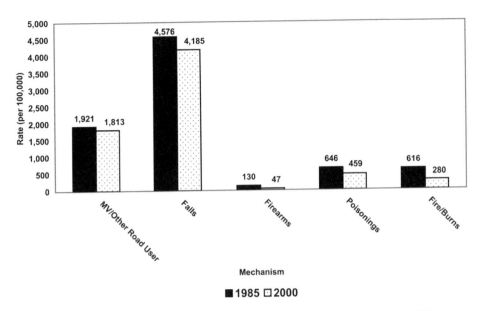

Figure 5.6 The Incidence Rate of Injuries (per 100,000) by Mechanism, 1985 vs. 2000

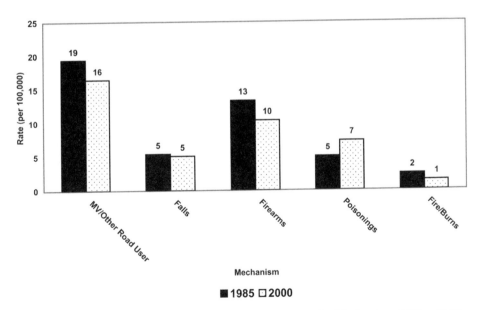

Figure 5.7 The Incidence Rate of Fatal Injuries (per 100,000) by Mechanism, 1985 vs. 2000

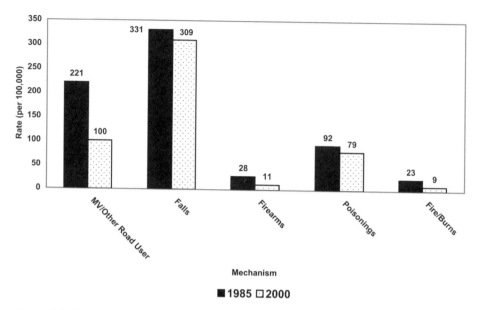

Figure 5.8 The Incidence Rate of Hospitalized Injuries (per 100,000) by Mechanism, 1985 vs. 2000

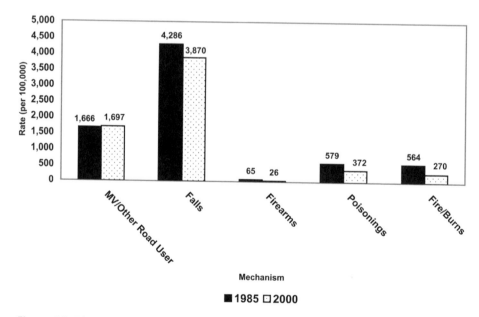

Figure 5.9 The Incidence Rate of Nonhospitalized Injuries (per 100,000) by Mechanism, 1985 vs. 2000

Table 5.3 The Incidence Rate of Injuries (per 100,000) by Age, Sex, and Mechanism, 1985 vs. 2000

	MV/Other Road User		Falls		Firearms		Poisonings		Fire/Burns	
	1985	2000	1985	2000	1985	2000	1985	2000	1985	2000
Male	*1,966*	*1,895*	*4,577*	*3,865*	*137*	*87*	*671*	*438*	*601*	*276*
0–4	627	720	7,400	7,388	2	5	1,996	1,089	819	661
5–14	957	1,733	6,612	5,716	72	143	654	68	381	127
15–24	3,780	3,392	4,321	3,176	220	197	453	431	824	433
25–44	2,418	2,374	3,159	2,660	246	87	654	528	787	266
45–64	1,590	1,323	3,347	2,639	48	34	525	351	257	260
65–74	958	969	4,872	3,934	41	27	512	662	515	95
75+	994	903	8,704	8,331	54	39	322	236	443	91
Female	*1,828*	*1,734*	*4,575*	*4,489*	*116*	*10*	*595*	*479*	*647*	*284*
0–4	743	440	7,612	5,885	2	2	1,869	463	600	427
5–14	1,116	1,338	6,645	4,561	94	10	661	246	105	127
15–24	2,966	3,353	4,794	2,978	116	23	250	1,309	612	228
25–44	2,329	2,168	3,485	2,988	256	11	558	356	1,195	178
45–64	1,221	1,362	2,894	4,137	10	7	431	192	394	512
65–74	1,234	1,181	3,206	5,120	5	4	597	1,244	259	316
75+	1,807	837	6,576	14,104	6	3	177	155	441	332

drownings/submersions (56%), and motor vehicle/other road users (55%). In contrast, the rate of hospitalized injuries for falls declined by a mere 6% from 1985 to 2000. For nonhospitalized injuries (Figure 5.9), the rate declined for all mechanisms with the exception of injuries sustained by motor vehicle/other road users. This most likely reflects the increased usage of safety belts and airbags, which served to decrease more serious injuries that resulted in hospitalization or death, while increasing minor injuries associated with the intervention itself (Chapter 1).

Table 5.3 shows the incidence rate of injuries by age, sex, and mechanism for 1985 and 2000. For motor-vehicle/other road-user injuries among males, rates declined only marginally for all age groups except those aged 0 to 14 years. For males aged 5 to 14 years, the rate of motor-vehicle/other road-user injuries nearly doubled from 1985 (957 per 100,000) to 2000 (1,733 per 100,000). For motor-vehicle/other road-user injuries among females, there were no consistent patterns of increase or decrease across age groups, however, the greatest rate of decline occurred among females aged 75 years and older (from 1,807 per 100,000 in 1985 to 837 per 100,000 in 2000).

For falls, the rate of injuries decreased for males in all age categories and for females in all age categories up to 45 years. In older females (aged 75 years and older), the rate of fall injuries more than doubled from 1985 (6,576 per 100,000 females) to 2000 (14,104 per 100,000). For firearms, the rate of injuries decreased from 1985 to 2000 for all age categories among females aged 5 years and older, and for all age categories among males aged 15 years and older. For poisonings, the rate of injuries marginally declined from 1985 to 2000 for most gender/age categories, with the exception of females aged 15 to 24 years (where the rate increased 5-fold) and females aged 65 to 74 years (where the rate increased 2-fold).

While the overall incidence of injuries declined by 15% from 1985 to 2000, the total medical costs of injuries (in real dollars) declined by roughly 20%. This decrease is driven in large part by the decrease in injury incidence, but may also be the result of advances in trauma care, a shift toward managed care and greater management of inpatient treatment, and successful injury prevention efforts (e.g., seatbelts, helmets) that minimize the harm resulting from injuries.

Implications for Prevention

The burden estimates provided in this book document the enormous toll that injuries impose on society. They also establish an estimated upper bound for determining savings that could be accrued through successful intervention efforts and can be used in cost-effectiveness and cost benefit analyses for targeted intervention efforts [Haddix et al. 2003]. Estimating the cost effectiveness or cost-benefit ratio of injury prevention strategies relative to other efforts aimed at improving health is useful to inform decisions about the allocation of scarce resources. The costs and outcomes of one intervention (e.g., child safety seat use), for example, can be compared with the costs and outcomes of another intervention (e.g., immunizations, drug abuse prevention) when the outcomes measured are the same, such as reductions in fatalities or dollars saved. Furthermore, trends in incidence and costs can spotlight specific populations where prevention efforts have been successful or where additional prevention efforts are needed.

The results presented in this text reveal that injuries continue to impose a significant health and financial burden on society. Although there are data limitations in interpreting the trends in incidence and medical costs presented here, the results suggest that several subpopulations could be considered for increased injury prevention efforts. Among the elderly, for example, particularly among elderly females, the incidence and costs of injuries are increasing, and much of this increase is due to falls. While evidence exists of effective and cost-effective strategies to prevent falls in the elderly (Chapter 1), widespread implementation of these effective interventions remains limited.

The trend data also highlight that motor-vehicle/other road-user injuries have significantly increased among males aged 5 to 14 years since 1985. Although supplementary research is required to identify the risk and protective factors associated with increased injuries in this population, effective prevention strategies (e.g., helmets, protective gear) are available and strategies for increasing access should be considered. One such strategy may be to subsidize the cost of the intervention (e.g., free or inexpensive bicycle helmets), especially if it is discovered by further research that motor-vehicle/other road-user injuries are more likely to occur among children living in low-income families who perhaps could not purchase the injury-prevention device at market prices. Because government is likely to bear a significant share of the medical cost of these injuries, it may be cost saving to subsidize a portion of the costs of the interventions. And because motor-vehicle/other road-user injuries among males are more likely to affect the young, who are more likely to have public sector health insurance (Table 5.3), subsidizing the costs for technology and risk-reduction programs among this population may also be cost saving.

The burden estimates also highlight areas where effective interventions may not yet be available. For example, poisoning injuries, which one might suspect are partially suicide-related, increased 5-fold from 1985 to 2000 among females aged 15 to 24 years. While some research examines the effectiveness and cost-effectiveness of secondary interventions designed to prevent suicidal re-attempts, less research addresses primary interventions designed to prevent suicide attempts from occurring in the first place. Similar gaps in prevention research are evident for other populations. For example, it is noteworthy that firearm injuries have doubled since 1985 among males aged 5 to 14 years. The burden of these injuries, which are substantial in terms of lives lost, pain and suffering, and economic consequences, should indicate to policy makers that this too is an area where more research is needed to find effective and cost-effective interventions targeting the prevention of injury that is both intentional and unintentional in nature.

Limitations

The lifetime costs of injuries in the United States reported in this book represent the best estimates available given existing data. However, as noted at the end of Chapters 1 through 3, important limitations are associated with both the incidence and cost estimates. As mentioned in these chapters, the ideal data source for calculating these estimates does not exist. As a result, we were forced to use myriad data sources, each with limitations. Some of these limitations include the age of the data, data based on nonnationally representative samples, and data subject to reporting and measurement error. This not only increases the lack of precision around the estimates but may result in additional bias. Although our approach was designed to minimize this bias, more current and nationally representative data would have been preferable.

Data that are missing include: (1) utilization and costs of mental-health services that were not identified as injury-related but were needed due to the psychological trauma of injury; (2) productivity losses for persons who were injured but did not seek medical treatment for their injuries; (3) productivity losses associated with the caregivers of injured persons (e.g., parents of injured children); and (4) utilization and costs of nontraditional health care services (e.g., chiropractors, acupuncturists, alternative medicine providers). The net effect of excluding these cases is likely to be substantial. For example, based on a survey of mental health providers, Cohen and Miller [1998] estimated that 3.4 million physical and sexual assaults resulted in mental health treatment, often without treatment in other medical settings. These treatment episodes are unlikely to be coded as injury related.

Data analyses that were not conducted include: (1) estimates of life years lost, quality-adjusted life years lost, or other losses in functional impairment; (2) stratification of the costs of injuries by payer (e.g., individual, government, private sector); (3) stratification of the incidence and cost of injuries by race, ethnicity, place of injury (e.g., workplace), or setting (e.g., rural, urban); and (4) stratification of the incidence and cost of injuries by intent (i.e., intentional, unintentional, war/legal, other). Data limitations and quality of existing data prevented us from conducting the first two analyses. While a stratification of injury incidence by race and ethnicity was possible, prevention efforts are not driven by these factors, therefore, we chose not to estimate incidence and costs by these strata.

Finally, we did not differentiate injuries by intent, and instead chose to combine unintentional injuries with those from intentional harm, such as child abuse and homicide. While stratifying results by intent is highly desirable for purposes of developing a prevention research agenda, we were concerned that reporting errors biased the results for intentional injuries downward. For example, many victims of intimate partner violence who seek medical attention for their injuries are more likely to self-identify the mechanism of the injury (e.g., a fall) without identifying the cause of the injury (e.g., pushed down the stairs by an intimate partner). One way to account for these reporting biases inherent in national surveillance and epidemiologic datasets is to supplement burden estimates found in analyses such as ours with other types of data collected in smaller in-person surveys and focus groups. Further research is needed in this area.

Concerning the productivity loss estimates, because women, the elderly, and children earn lower wages, the human capital approach undervalues injuries to these groups. The approach also places lower values on the work of full-time homemakers than the work of people participating in the labor market, which might further depress the value placed on women's productivity losses relative to men's productivity losses.

An additional limitation of both this text and the 1989 report to Congress [Rice et al. 1989] is the lack of standard errors. The estimates generated from this (and their) analysis are associated with uncertainty, and readers are cautioned that the actual incidence or costs for a given injury category could be higher or lower than what is reported here. As a result, comparisons across strata and over time should be interpreted with caution.

The comparisons to the 1989 report to Congress include additional caveats. Different data sources were used for some of the analyses. Most of the current data sources are better in terms of the injury information captured (e.g., type, nature, severity) and cost data available, but some of the same sources collect different or less information than before. For example, the incidence estimates published in the original report included injuries that resulted in lost workdays and/or bed days for which no medical treatment was sought. This information is no longer collected in currently available data sources. Therefore, to allow us to make a fair comparison between the 2000 and 1985 incidence estimates, we reduced the 1985 incidence estimates to focus solely on injuries receiving medical attention, using data provided by the authors of that report.

A direct comparison of medical costs may be problematic as differences in costs could be driven by the inflation factor used for the analysis, differences in cost to charge ratios over time, and other market-based factors that would influence costs independent of changes in treatment patterns. Moreover, while we can make a general comparison of the burden sustained by lifetime medical costs from 1985 to 2000, we cannot similarly compare the burden of productivity losses. In particular, differences in how productivity losses were calculated (i.e., discount rate, annual growth rate in income) are factors that prevent this comparison.

Despite these limitations, the data in this book provide unequivocal evidence of the large health and financial burden of injuries. Policy makers have the ability to influence this burden through legislation, money, support, direct implementation of injury prevention efforts, research, advocacy, and other mechanisms. All of these strategies should be considered in efforts to reduce the burden that injuries impose on society.

Works Cited

Ahrens M. *U.S. Experience with Smoke Alarms and Other Fire Alarms.* Quincy, Mass: National Fire Protection Association; 2001.

American Geriatrics Society, British Geriatrics Society, American Academy of Orthopaedic Surgeons Panel on Falls Prevention. Guideline for the prevention of falls in older persons. *Journal of the American Geriatrics Society.* 2001;49(5):664–672.

Aos S, Phipps P, Barnoski R, Lieb R. *The Comparative Costs and Benefits of Programs to Reduce Crime, Version 4.0.* Seattle, Wash: Washington State Institute for Public Policy; 2001. 01-05-1201.

Arias E. United States life tables, 2000. *National Vital Statistics Reports.* Vol 51. Hyattsville, Md: National Center for Health Statistics; 2002.

Berkowitz M, Harvey C, Greene C, Wilson S. *The Economic Consequences of Spinal Cord Injury.* Washington, DC: Paralysis Society of America of the Paralyzed Veterans of America; 1990.

Branche CM, Stewart S. *Lifeguard Effectiveness: A Report of the Working Group.* Atlanta, Ga: Centers for Disease Control and Prevention, National Center for Injury Prevention and Control; 2001.

Brenner RA, Trumble AC, Smith GS, Kessler EP, Overpeck MD. Where children drown, United States, 1995. *Pediatrics.* 2001;108(1):85–89.

Bureau of Labor Statistics. *Highlights of Women's Earnings in 2000.* Washington, DC: Bureau of Labor Statistics; 2001. BLS Report 952.

Bureau of the Census. *US Statistical Abstract.* Washington, DC: Bureau of the Census; 2002.

Butcher JL, MacKenzie EJ, Cushing B, et al. Long-term outcomes after lower extremity trauma. *Journal of Trauma.* 1996;41(1):4–9.

Centers for Disease Control and Prevention. Motor vehicle safety: a 20th century public health success. *Morbidity and Mortality Weekly Report.* 1999;48(18):369–374.

Centers for Disease Control and Prevention. Community interventions to promote healthy social environments: Early childhood development and family housing. A report on recommendations of the task force on community preventive services. *Morbidity and Mortality Weekly Report.* 2002;51(RR01):1–8.

Centers for Disease Control and Prevention. First reports evaluating the effectiveness of strategies for preventing violence: early childhood home visitation and firearms laws. Findings from the Task Force on Community Preventive Services. *Morbidity and Mortality Weekly Report.* 2003;52(RR-14):1–9.

Centers for Disease Control and Prevention. Unintentional and undetermined poisoning deaths—11 states, 1990–2001. *Morbidity and Mortality Weekly Report.* 2004;53(11): 233–238.

Centers for Disease Control and Prevention. Web-based injury statistics query and reporting system (WISQARS). *National Center for Injury Prevention and Control, Centers for Disease Control and Prevention* [online]. Available at: www.cdc.gov/ncipc/wisqars. Accessed September 17, 2004.

Clemson L, Cumming RG, Kendig H, Swann M, Heard R, Taylor K. The effectiveness of a community-based program for reducing the incidence of falls in the elderly: a randomized trial. *Journal of the American Geriatrics Society.* 2004;52(9):1487–1494.

Close J, Ellis M, Hooper R, Glucksman E, Jackson S, Swift C. Prevention of falls in the elderly trial (PROFET): a randomised controlled trial. *Lancet.* 1999;353(9147):93–97.

Cohen MA, Miller TR. The cost of mental health care for victims of crime. *Journal of Interpersonal Violence.* 1998;13(1):93–110.

Cummings P, Grossman DC, Rivara FP, Koepsell TD. State gun safe storage laws and child mortality due to firearms. *Journal of the American Medical Association.* 1997;278(13): 1084–1086.

Davis MA, Neuhaus JM, Moritz DJ, Lein D, Barclay JD, Murphy SP. Health behaviors and survival among middle aged and older men and women in the NHANES I Epidemiologic Follow-Up Study. *Preventative Medicine.* 1994;23(3):369–376.

Day L, Fildes B, Gordon I, Fitzharris M, Flamer H, Lord S. Randomised factorial trial of falls prevention among older people living in their own homes. *British Medical Journal.* 2002;325(7356):128.

Dellinger A, Sleet D, Jones B. Motor vehicle safety. In: Ward J, ed. *A Safer, Healthier America: The Advancement of Public Health in the 20th Century.* London: Oxford University Press; 2005, in press.

Dikmen SS, Temkin NR, Machamer JE, Holubkov AL, Fraser RT, Winn HR. Employment following traumatic head injuries. *Archives of Neurology.* 1994;51(2):177–186.

Durlack JA. Health promotion as a strategy for primary prevention. In: Cicchetti D, Rappaport J, Sandler I, Weissberg RP, eds. *The Promotion of Wellness in Children and Adolescents.* Washington, DC: CWLA Press; 2000:221–241.

Eber GB, Annest JL, Mercy JA, Ryan GW. Nonfatal and fatal firearm-related injuries among children aged 14 years and younger: United States, 1993–2000. *Pediatrics.* 2004;113(6): 1686–1692.

Edwards CM, Mackintosh DR, Claid D. *Patient Cost and Economic Burden due to Accidental Injuries.* Washington, DC: National Institute for Advanced Studies; 1981. Final report submitted to the Center for Environmental Health, CDC, under Contract 200-79-0964.

Englander J, Hall K, Stimpson T, Chaffin S. Mild traumatic brain injury in an insured population: subjective complaints and return to employment. *Brain Injury.* 1992;6(2):161–166.

Finkelstein EA, Fiebelkorn IA, Corso PS, Binder SC. Medical expenditures attributable to injuries—United States, 2000. *Morbidity and Mortality Weekly Report.* 2004;53(1):1–4.

Foshee VA, Bauman KE, Ennett ST, Linder GF, Benefield T, Suchindran C. Assessing the long-term effects of the Safe Dates program and a booster in preventing and reducing adolescent dating violence victimization and perpetration. *American Journal of Public Health.* 2004;94(4):619–624.

Friedman B, De La Mare J, Andrews R, McKenzie DH. Practical options for estimating cost of hospital inpatient stays. *Journal of Health Care Finance.* 2002;29(1):1–13.

Gilchrist J, Gotsch K, Ryan GW. Nonfatal and fatal drownings in recreational water settings—United States, 2001–2002. *Morbidity and Mortality Weekly Report.* 2004;53(21): 447–452.

Gillespie LD, Gillespie WJ, Robertson MC, Lamb SE, Cumming RG, Rowe BH. Interventions for preventing falls in elderly people (Cochrane review). *The Cochrane Library, Issue 3.* Oxford: Update Software; 2002.

Gillespie LD, Gillespie WJ, Robertson MC, Lamb SE, Cumming RG, Rowe BH. Interventions for preventing falls in elderly people (Cochrane review). *The Cochrane Library, Issue 3, 2004.* Chichester, UK: John Wiley & Sons, Ltd.; 2004.

Goldsmith SK, Pellmar TC, Kleinman AM, Bunney WE. *Reducing Suicide: A National Imperative.* Washington, DC: The National Academies Press; 2002.

Greenspan SL, Myers ER, Maitland LA, Kido TH, Krasnow MB, Hayes WC. Trochanteric bone mineral density is associated with type of hip fracture in the elderly. *Journal of Bone and Mineral Research.* 1994;9(12):1889–1894.

Grossman DC, Cummings P, Koepsell TD, et al. Firearm safety counseling in primary care pediatrics: a randomized, controlled trial. *Pediatrics.* 2000;106(1 Pt 1):22–26.

Grossman DC, Mueller BA, Riedy C, et al. Gun storage practices and risk of youth suicide and unintentional firearm injuries. *Journal of the American Medical Association.* 2005;293(6): 707–714.

Grossman JB, Garry EM. *Mentoring: A Proven Delinquency Prevention Strategy.* Washington, DC: U. S. Department of Justice, Office of Justice Programs; 1997. (Juvenile Justice Bulletin, No. NCJ 164386.

Haddix AC, Teutsch SM, Corso PS. *Prevention Effectiveness: A Guide to Decision Analysis and Economic Evaluation.* 2nd ed. New York, NY: Oxford University Press; 2003.

Hall JR. *Burns, Toxic Gases, and Other Hazards Associated with Fires: Deaths and Injuries in Fire and Non-fire Situations.* Quincy, Mass: National Fire Protection Association, Fire Analysis and Research Division; 2001.

Hardy MS. Behavior-oriented approaches to reducing youth gun violence. *Future of Children.* 2002;12(2):100–117.

Hausdorff JM, Rios DA, Edelberg HK. Gait variability and fall risk in community-living older adults: a 1-year prospective study. *Archives of Physical Medicine and Rehabilitation.* 2001;82(8):1050–1056.

Hill K, et al. *An Analysis of Research on Preventing Falls and Falls Injury in Older People: Community, Residential Aged Care and Acute Care Settings (2004 update).* Commonwealth of Australia: Health and Aged Care, National Aging Research Institute; 2004.

Hill K, Smith R, Murray K, et al. *An Analysis of Research on Preventing Falls and Falls Injury in Older People: Community, Residential Aged Care and Acute Care Settings.* Canberra, Australia: National Ageing Research Institute, Centre for Applied Gerontology; 2000.

Hodgson T, Meiners M. Cost-of-illness methodology: a guide to current practices and procedures. *Milbank Memorial Fund Quarterly.* 1982;60(3):429–462.

Hornbrook MC, Stevens VJ, Wingfield DJ, Hollis JF, Greenlick MR, Ory MG. Preventing falls among community-dwelling older persons: results from a randomized trial. *The Gerontologist.* 1994;34(1):16–23.

Hornick JP, Paetsch JJ, Bertrand LD. *A Manual on Conducting Economic Analysis of Crime Prevention Programs.* Ottawa, Ontario: National Crime Prevention Centre; 2000.

Howland J, Hingson R. Alcohol as a risk factor for drownings: a review of the literature (1950–1985). *Accident Analysis and Prevention.* 1988;20(1):19–25.

Howland J, Mangione T, Hingson R, Smith G, Bell N. Alcohol as a risk factor for drowning and other aquatic injuries. In: Watson RR, ed. *Alcohol and Accidents. Drug and Alcohol Abuse Reviews.* Vol 7. Totowa, NJ: Humana Press, Inc.; 1995.

Istre GR, McCoy MA, Osborn L, Barnard JJ, Bolton A. Deaths and injuries from house fires. *New England Journal of Medicine.* 2001;344(25):1911–1916.

Kalafat J. Issues in the evaluation of youth suicide prevention initiatives. In: Joiner T, Rudd MD, eds. *Suicide Science: Expanding the Boundaries.* Boston, Mass: Kluwer Academic Publishers; 2000:241–249.

Karter MJ. *Fire Loss in the United States during 2003.* Quincy, Mass: National Fire Protection Association, Fire Analysis and Research Division; 2004.

Knox KL, Litts DA, Talcott GW, Feig JC, Caine ED. Risk of suicide and related adverse outcomes after exposure to a suicide prevention programme in the US Air Force: cohort study. *British Medical Journal.* 12/13 2003;327(7428):1376.

Lambert MT, Silva PS. An update on the impact of gun control legislation on suicide. *The Psychiatric Quarterly.* 1998;69(2):127–134.

Lawrence BA, Miller TR, Jensen AF, Fisher DA, Zamula WW. Estimating the costs of non-fatal consumer product injuries in the United States. *Injury Control & Safety Promotion—2000.* 2000;7(2):97–113.

Loftin C, McDowall D, Wiersema B, Cottey TJ. Effects of restrictive licensing of handguns on homicide and suicide in the District of Columbia. *New England Journal of Medicine.* 1991;325:1615–1620.

Ludwig J, Duncan GJ, Hirschfield P. Urban poverty and juvenile crime: evidence from a randomized housing-mobility experiment. *Quarterly Journal of Economics.* 2001;16:655–680.

MacKenzie EJ, Siegel JH, Shapiro S, Moody M, Smith RT. Functional recovery and medical costs of trauma: an analysis by type and severity of injury. *Journal of Trauma.* 1988;28(3):281–297.

McMurdo ME, Millar AM, Daly F. A randomized controlled trial of fall prevention strategies in old peoples' homes. *Gerontology.* 2000;46(2):83–87.

Melton LJ, Chrischilles EA, Cooper C, Lane AW, Riggs BL. How many women have osteoporosis? *Journal of Bone and Mineral Research.* 1992;7(9):1005–1010.

Mercy JA, Butchart A, Farrington D, Cerda M. Youth violence. In: Krug EG, Dahlberg LL, Mercy JA, Zwi AB, Lozano R, eds. *World Report on Violence and Health.* Geneva, Switzerland: World Health Organization; 2002:25–56.

Michel K, Frey C, Wyss K, Valach L. An exercise in improving suicide reporting in print media. *Crisis.* 2000;21(2):71–79.

Miller TR, Brigham P, Cohen M, et al. Estimating the costs to society of cigarette fire injuries. *Report to Congress in Response to the Fire Safe Cigarette Act of 1990.* Vol 85. Washington, DC: U.S. Government Printing Office and Consumer Product Safety Commission; 1993:932–938.

Miller TR, Cohen MA. Costs of gunshot and cut/stab wounds in the United States, with some Canadian comparisons. *Accident Analysis and Prevention.* 1997;29(3):329–341.

Miller TR, Ireland TR. Emerging issues in estimating lifetime costs: life tables and productivity losses. In: Luchter S, MacKenzie EJ, eds. *Measuring the Burden of Injury, 3rd International Conference Proceedings.* Baltimore, MD: National Highway Traffic Safety Administration; 2000:88–93.

Miller TR, Langston EA, Lawrence BA, et al. *Rehabilitation Costs and Long-Term Consequences of Motor Vehicle Injury.* Calverton, Md: Pacific Institute for Research and Evaluation; 2004. Final report to National Highway Traffic Safety Administration.

Miller TR, Levy D. Cost-outcome analysis in injury prevention and control: a primer on methods. *Injury Prevention.* 1997;3(4):288–293.

Miller TR, Pindus NM, Douglass JB, Rossman SB. *Databook on Nonfatal Injury: Incidence, Costs, and Consequences.* Washington, DC: The Urban Institute Press; 1995.

Miller TR, Romano ED, Spicer RS. The cost of childhood unintentional injuries and the value of prevention. *The Future of Children.* 2000;10(1):137–163.

Morris JAJ, Sanchez AA, Bass SM, MacKenzie EJ. Trauma patients return to productivity. *Journal of Trauma.* 06/01 1991;31(6):827–833; discussion 833–834.

National Center for Injury Prevention and Control. *Costs of Intimate Partner Violence Against Women in the United States.* Atlanta, Ga: Centers for Disease Control and Prevention; 2003.

National Highway Traffic Safety Administration. *Economic Cost of Motor Vehicle Crashes, 2000.* Washington, DC: National Highway Traffic Safety Administration; 2002.

National Pediatric Trauma Registry. *Biannual Report, December 2001.* Boston, Mass: Tufts University; 2002.

National Research Council. Firearms and violence: a critical review. In: Wellford CF, Pepper JV, Petrie CV, eds. *Committee on Law and Justice, Division of Behavioral and Social Sci-*

ences and Education. Committee to Improve Research Information and Data on Firearms ed. Washington, DC: The National Academies Press; 2005.

National Safety Council. *Injury Facts.* Itasca, IL: National Safety Council; 2003.

Nikolaus T, Bach M. Preventing falls in community-dwelling frail older people using a home intervention team (HIT): results from the randomized Falls-HIT trial. *Journal of the American Geriatrics Society.* 2003;51(3):300–305.

Owens DK. Analytic tools for public health decision making. *Medical Decision Making.* 2002;22(5 Suppl):S3–S10.

Parks T, Usdin S, Goldstein S. Health promotion, violence prevention and the media: the Soul City campaign. In: Krug EG, Dahlberg LL, Mercy JA, Zwi AB, Lozano R, eds. *World Report on Violence and Health.* Geneva, Switzerland; 2002:250.

Peden M, Scurfield R, Sleet D, et al. *World Report on Road Traffic Injury Prevention.* Geneva, Switzerland: World Health Organization; 2004.

Public Health Service. *National Strategy for Suicide Prevention: Goals and Objectives.* Rockville, Md: U.S. Department of Health and Human Services; 2001.

RAND, Southern California Evidence-Based Practice Center. *Evidence Report and Evidence-Based Recommendations: Fall Prevention Interventions in the Medicare Population.* Baltimore, Md: U.S. Department of Health and Human Services, Centers for Medicare & Medicaid Services; 2003.

Rice DP. Estimating the cost of illness. *U.S. Public Health Economics Series (No. 6).* Washington, DC: U.S. Public Health Service (PHS No. 947–6); 1966.

Rice DP. Estimating the cost of illness. *American Journal of Public Health Nations Health.* 1967;57(3):424–440.

Rice DP, Hodgson TA, Kopstein AN. The economics of illness: a replication and update. *Health Care Financing Review.* 1985;7:61–80.

Rice DP, MacKenzie EJ, Jones AS, et al. *Cost of Injury in the United States: A Report to Congress.* San Francisco, Calif: Institute for Health & Aging, University of California, and Injury Prevention Center, The Johns Hopkins University; 1989.

Ruffolo CF, Friedland JF, Dawson DR, Colantonio A, Lindsay PH. Mild traumatic brain injury from motor vehicle accidents: factors associated with return to work. *Archives of Physical Medicine and Rehabilitation.* 1999;80(4):392–398.

Scott VJ, Dukeshire S, Gallagher EM, Scanlan A. *A Best Practices Guide for the Prevention of Falls Among Seniors Living in the Community.* Ottawa, Ontario: Minister of Public Works and Government Services; 2001.

Shaffer D, Garland A, Gould M, Fisher P, Trautman P. Preventing teenage suicide: a critical review. *Journal of the American Academy of Child and Adolescent Psychiatry.* 1988;27(6):675–687.

Smith GS, Branas CC, Miller TR. Fatal nontraffic injuries involving alcohol: a meta-analysis. *Annals of Emergency Medicine.* 1999;33(6):659–668.

Sterling DA, O'Connor JA, Bonadies J. Geriatric falls: Injury severity is high and disproportionate to mechanism. *Journal of Trauma-Injury Infection and Critical Care.* 2001;50(1):116–119.

Teret SP, Culross PL. Product-oriented approaches to reducing youth gun violence. *Future of Children.* 2002;12(2):118–131.

Thompson EA, Eggert LL, Randell BP, Pike KC. Evaluation of indicated suicide risk prevention approaches for potential high school dropouts. *American Journal of Public Health.* 2001;91(5):742–752.

Thornhill S, Teasdale GM, Murray GD, McEwen J, Roy CW, Penny KI. Disability in young people and adults one year after head injury: prospective cohort study. *British Medical Journal.* 2000;320(7250):1631–1635.

United Nations Population Fund. UNFPA annual report, 1998: reproductive health effects of gender-based violence. *United Nations Population Fund (UNFPA)* [Online]. Available at: http://www.unfpa.org/about/report/report98/ppgenderbased.htm. Accessed January 15, 2005.

United States Fire Administration, Federal Emergency Management Agency, National Fire

Data Center. *Fire in the United States: 1989–1998.* Emmitsburg, Md: United States Fire Administration; 2001. 12th ed.

U.S. Census Bureau. Table 713. Consumer price indexes (COI-U) by major groups: 1980 to 2002. *Statistical Abstract of the United States: 2003.* Washington, DC: U.S. Census Bureau; 2003:475.

U.S. Coast Guard. Boating statistics—2002. *U.S. Department of Homeland Security, United States Coast Guard* [Online]. Available at: http://www.uscgboating.org/statistics/accident_stats.htm. Accessed February 24, 2004.

U.S. Consumer Product Safety Commission. *CPSC Staff Recommendations for Barriers for Residential Swimming Pools, Spas, and Hot Tubs.* Washington, DC: United States Consumer Product Safety Commission; 1991.

U.S. Department of Health and Human Services. *Youth Violence: A Report of the Surgeon General.* Rockville, Md: U.S. Department of Health and Human Services, Centers for Disease Control and Prevention, National Center for Injury Prevention and Control; Substance Abuse and Mental Health Services Administration, Center for Mental Health Services; and National Institutes of Health, National Institute of Mental Health; 2001.

Utting D. Prevention through family and parenting programs. In: Farrington DP, Coid JW, eds. *Early Prevention of Adult Antisocial Behaviour.* Cambridge, Mass: Cambridge University Press; 2003:243–264.

Wainer H. Robust statistics: a survey and some prescriptions. *Journal of Educational Statistics.* 1976;1(4):285–312.

Zaloshnja E, Miller T, Romano E, Spicer R. Crash costs by body part injured, fracture involvement, and threat to life severity, United States, 2000. *Accident Analysis and Prevention.* May 2004;36(3):415–427.

Index